Essential Oils

Discover "Anti-Aging" Remedies & Beauty Secrets:

Your Complete Wellness Guide to Body Care, Skin Care & Aromatherapy

New and Improved – 3rd Edition

By: Gabriel E. Wise

1

5

Table of Contents

Introduction

Mainstream skin and body care products aren't for everyone. In fact, they are often full of so many processed ingredients that they cause more problems than they solve. If you have been interested in learning about how you can use essential oils to create your skin and body care products at home or if you are looking for a larger variety of things that can be done with your essential oils, this book is going to provide the information you are looking for.

Starting with a brief lesson on what essentials are, how to use them and some precautions that you should know before investing in any essential oils, this book is going to go much deeper. This book is going to go into depth on the best essential oils for many different beauty problems that people face, as well as essential oils that cater to the many different skin types that people can have.

Aging is a natural part of life but one that often happens earlier in our life than we would like it to. Wrinkles, scars, stretch marks and varicose veins are all things that can be lightened and reversed with the use of essential oils, and this book is going to show you which essential oils are best for each of these applications.

We aren't going to stop there. We are also going to cover hair care, as well as some other applications for essential oils including using them to relieve the effects of depression, anxiety and many common coughs, cold and sinus symptoms.

Did you know that everything you use around the house could affect your health? This book is also going to have a look at some of the products you are using around your house and how you can replace those products with homemade products using essential oils. The things you can do with essential oils are limitless, and this book is going to explore many of the options that are available to you!

This book is laid out in easy to read chapters that are loaded with the information you are looking for when it comes to essential oils and numerous recipes that show all the ways they can be used.

Before we begin, here is a small GIFT, a BONUS book from my publisher as a thank you for buying this book.

The Ultimate Salad Recipe Collection

More than 350 easy-to-follow recipes, including both classic favorites and fresh new ideas.

Inside you'll find salads designed to suit any occasion throughout the year -- from a summer barbecue to an elegant dinner with family or friends.

Just go to the below link to get it -

https://shininguniverseenergy.leadpages.co/ultimate-salad-recipe/

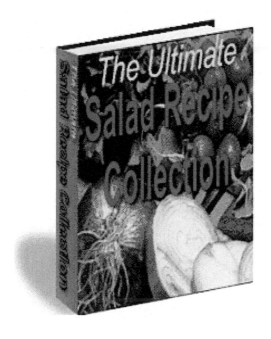

Hope you like your GIFT. Let's now learn about Essential Oils.

Chapter 1: A Quick Lesson on Essential Oils

Before we delve into what essential oils can do for you, we are going to take a quick minute to explain what exactly essential oils are, how they are made and how to choose your essential oils. This is going to help you later on when you are creating your recipes to make sure you have the foundation you need to understand fully how those recipes are going to work for you.

What Are Essential Oils?

The term "essential oil" stems from the original term "quintessential oil." This dates back to the Aristotelian idea that all matter is composed of four elements: fire, water, earth and air. Quintessence was considered to be a fifth element that was deemed to be the spirit or life force. Evaporation and Distillation were thought to be processes which removed the spirit from the plant. This reflects in our modern day language where we use the term spirits to describe beverages such as whiskey and brandy.

An essential oil is an oil that occurs naturally in a plant or other source. It is typically obtained by distillation and has the characteristic fragrance of the plant it was extracted from.

How Are Essential Oils Made?

Essential oils are extracted through two methods: distillation and expression.

Distillation:

It is thought that aromatic oils have been extracted through the practice of steam distillation for the last 5000 years. It is still the more common practice of extracting essential oils from plants because the components can be distilled at temperatures that are lower than their boiling points and are easily separated from the condensed water. There are three different types of distillation, although the basics of the distillation process are the same regardless of which method is used.

During distillation, the plant material is placed on a grid inside the still, which is the apparatus that is used to extract the oils. Once the plant is inside, the still is sealed and then depending on the extraction method being used, steam or water/steam is used to slowly break down the plant material to remove its volatile constituents or the aromatic extract. The volatile constituents rise upwards towards a pipe that leads them into a condenser which cools the vapor and turns it back into a liquid. The liquid will then be collected in a vehicle below the condenser. Since, like any oil, essential oils and water do not mix, the essential oil will be found on top of the water and siphoned off. Occasionally, the oil is heavier than the water, such as with clove essential oil and will be found at the bottom of the water.

The Three Types of Distillation

1. **Water Distillation**: During water distillation, the plant material comes into direct contact with

the water. This method is commonly used when extracting from flowers, such as rose and orange blossoms because steam causes these flowers to clump together which prevents steam from passing through.

2. **Water and Steam Distillation**: Water and Steam distillation is common with herb and leaf material. During water and steam distillation, the water remains below the plant material that is placed on the grate while steam is introduced from outside the main still.

3. **Steam Distillation**: During steam distillation, steam is injected into the still at a pressure and temperature that is slightly higher than water or water and steam distillation. Steam distillation is most commonly used for extraction.

Expression:

Also referred to as cold pressing, Expression is a method of extraction that is unique to citrus essential oils. Some of the oils that would use the expression extraction method are lemon, sweet orange, tangerine, bergamot, and lime. While expression used to be done by hand, we use a more modern, less labor intensive process today. During the process of expression, the rind of the fruit is placed into a container that has spikes that will puncture the fruit rind as the device is rotated. This technique is accomplished using centrifugal force. The spinning and puncturing release the essential oil that is then collected in a small area below the container. Spinning in a centrifugal force causes most of the essential oil to separate from the fruit juice.

DIY Extraction of Essential Oils

It is easy to extract essential oils from different parts of plants at home using the simplest techniques. This section explains these techniques in detail. These methods are easy and don't require too much preparation.

Extraction of oils using oil:

You may be wondering how one can extract oils using oil. This section entails the process you would need to follow. This extraction process is based on the assumption that oils attract oils. It is easier to extract the oils from the plants and the flowers using oil, based on this assumption. All you need to do is soak the parts of the herbs you want to extract oil from in oil. Let us take a look at the procedure to follow.

1. Take a non - metal container and pour olive oil into it. Make sure you pour enough oil to cover the herbs and plants that you are going to place into the pot.

2. Put in the leaves or the flowers of the plant whose oil you would like to extract.

3. Set the container aside for two days.

4. Strain the mixture of the oil and herbs by pressing the leaves and the flowers gently. This will help to release more oils.

5. Now add more of the leaves and flowers of the plant. Repeat the above steps.

6. You will need to continue to perform these steps until you have obtained essential oil that is rich.

7. Store the oil in a dark place. Make sure that the vial or the bottle you use to store the oil is sealed well.

Extracting oils using alcohol:

This is another simple technique that can be used to extract essential oils. You have to soak the leaves and the flowers of the plant whose oil you would like to extract in alcohol. The only alcohol that can be used in this process is undenatured ethyl alcohol. You can use vodka if you cannot find the ethyl alcohol, but try to avoid using rubbing alcohol.

The process followed is the same process used to extract using oil. You can either use the alcohol in its pure form, or you can dilute it with water. The extracts that you make using alcohol are as perfect as perfumes.

When you need to separate the oil from alcohol, leave the bowl in the deep freeze. This will ensure that the oil solidifies at the top of the bowl. The oil does not freeze and can be grazed off. You could use this for delicate flowers like jasmine since this process does not burn the petals off.

Choosing Essential Oils

Many people today tend to be frugal and want to stretch their dollar as far as they can. However, this isn't always the best idea when it comes to essential oils. As you can see from the description on how essential oils are produced, it takes a lot of a plant to make a small amount of the oil. It stands to reason that essential oils, at least pure essential oils are going to be pricier.

In fact, to make one pound of the essential oil lavender, it takes one hundred pounds of the lavender plant. On a more extreme end, it takes four thousand pounds of Bulgarian roses to make just one pound of the essential oil.

Why Pure Essential Oils Are Better:

Before getting too far into explaining how to choose your essential oils, let's take a look at why you should always choose pure essential oils over blends. Perhaps the biggest reason you want to select pure essential oils over blends is that they are going to work better. Blended oils often don't achieve the same desired effect as pure oils do in the recipes that they are used in.

**Things to Consider When Choosing Your
Essential Oil Supplier**:

You can find essential oils in most stores that have a pharmacy section. You can also find them in whole food stores and online. However, there are a few things you are going to want to consider when you are deciding on a supplier/company to buy from. It is important to choose a supplier/company that:

- Is smaller over a large corporation

- Is owned by an aromatherapy practitioner or an essential oil specialist

- Have relations with his/her distillers

- Can provide data sheets on the material safety when needed

28

- Can supply a specification report that is batch specific for each essential oil it sells

- Doesn't promote the unsafe use of essential oils

- Doesn't sell essential oils of plants that are endangered

- Has a good reputation

- Has been in the business of essential oils for many years

If you want to test your essential oil to see how "pure" it is, there is a simple test you can do. Put a single drop of the essential oil onto a piece of construction paper. If it quickly evaporates and doesn't leave a noticeable ring, it is pure. If there is a ring left behind, it was likely diluted by the manufacturer with an oil of some sort. Keep in mind this test is not accurate with myrrh, patchouli, and absolutes.

Something you should consider when comparing the prices of essential oils is that essential oils that are listed as "not for internal consumption" are going to be less expensive than others that aren't labeled as such. The reason for the "not for consumption" labels is that the only way to avoid that label is to spend hundreds of millions of dollars on insurance and training. The companies that label their essential oils as "not for internal consumption" save money on insurance and provide their essential oils for a lower price.

If you are shopping for essential oils and you come across a label that says "fragrance" or "fragrance oil" or even "perfume" anywhere, you can assume that this is a synthetic product and not a natural product. This is true even if it says that it is a natural fragrance. A natural fragrance is not the same thing as an essential oil, and good, high quality essential oils do not include fragrance or fragrance oil of any kind.

Uses of Essential Oils

Use in Pharmacology:

There are a lot of people skeptical towards the use of essential oils in healthcare and pharmacy produce. However, these oils have been used extensively in fringe medicine and also in popular medicine for a long time. After thorough research had been conducted on essential oils, it was proved that oils have properties that allow them to prevent the transmission of pathogens like Staphylococcus and Candid. These pathogens are drug resistant.

Since these oils are highly concentrated, they cannot be taken directly by mouth. If one does take it by mouth, he might have a burning sensation, which is followed by increased salivation. There may be more gas that is released in the stomach, which may induce eructation or belching. It has been found that the effect is antispasmodic in your intestines.

It has been found that essential oils like eucalyptus oil and menthol are great ingredients for medicines to be used externally. Other oils can be utilized too, but they do not have any special properties and benefits. This proves that the oils can be used differently based on their pharmacology. Some essential oils might be perfect for the upper part of your body – respiratory tract, stomach; while some might be better for your lower body. Some oils can also be used as anesthetics. Some oils, like the oil of juniper, have been used for their properties as diuretics. There have been many concerns raised by the extensive use of antibacterial agents. Essential oils have now become a substitute for these agents. They are also being tested clinically to understand the extent to which their properties can be used.

Quite a few essential oils affect the skin and the membranes in a helpful way. However, if used in excess, it might harm the skin. Certain essential oils irritate and then help in reducing the pain and irritation by creating a feeling of numbness. Some are used as antiseptics and local anesthetics. Thymol is an excellent example of an essential oil used as an antiseptic.

Use in Aromatherapy:

Aromatherapy is a branch of medicine that is based on the fact that the aromatic properties of the oils have healing effects on the body and the mind. There have been many writings that prove that essential oils have been used in the form of folk medicine since ancient times. These oils are still widely used because of their medicinal properties. It has been claimed that these oils have a significant effect on the mind. They help in relieving stress and also assist in calming the mind down. The uses of essential oils and the benefits of Aromatherapy have been explained in detail in Chapter 20.

General Uses:

There are numerous ways in which essential oils can be used around the house. This section covers a few of those uses.

Uses for the body and mind

- You can use essential oils to make your very own scrub packs. You will need to dilute them to ensure that they do not harm your skin. The most common scrub is the salt scrub, which is made using almond oil. This helps in making your skin incredibly soft to touch.

- Essential oils can be used during baths, and also in body lotions. When you pour a few drops of essential oils into your bath, you will find that the bath smells immensely fresh and you come out feeling very clean. Essential oils make you relax and feel calm after a hectic day at work. You can mix a few drops of essential oils in a bottle of organic coconut oil. This works as a body lotion and keeps your skin smooth and rejuvenated.

- It is advisable to pour a few drops of essential oil onto your handkerchief and place it under your pillow. This is an idea based on aromatherapy. It is found that the aromatic component of the oil helps in relaxing and calming the mind. You find that you have a better sleep and better dreams.

- Perfumes are expensive, and those with brand names may be out of your budget. They cost a whopping amount of money. It would be easy if we could make our very own perfumes at home would it not? It is a simple mixture. Use a few floral scents, something you might like – maybe rose or lily. Add a few drops of Jojoba Oil to the scent. You can apply this with ease on your skin since it does not cause any irritation. It also smells wonderful, and the scent lasts all day! You can also rub a few drops of the oil of vanilla behind your ears. This oil is the least harmful and can be used on the skin without worrying.

- You can also use essential oils in your lip balm. These days, every lip balm comes with a few essential oils as part of the ingredients. It has been found that essential oils in these lotions make our lips smooth and soft to touch.

Household Uses

- You can always use essential oils to refresh the furniture at home. Fill half a bottle with hot water, the other half with vinegar and add a few slices of lime to the bottle. Now add a few drops of lavender and clove oils! Your furniture looks brand new once again!

- You can use essential oils in your laundry detergent. This leaves your clothes smelling like heaven!

- Essential oils can be used in disinfectants. It has been found that essential oils like tea tree oil have excellent disinfectant properties and help remove bacteria and fungus. You can use this oil as a disinfectant.

- If you have carpets at home, you find that they need to be vacuumed regularly to avoid an attack from fleas. You can make your life easier by using essential oils. You can use tea tree oil and other essential oils. Mix a few drops of this oil with Borax to make your very own flea powder.

- Did you know you could use essential oils as bug repellents? Yes, surprising is it not? You can mix a few drops of essential oils into a bottle of hot water and spray it around the

37

house. It is very safe to use around children as well!

- Cleaning sprays are full of chemicals and cannot be used in a house with children. Instead, you can use Pine Needle essential oil. Add a few drops of this oil to a bottle of water and put that in a large spray bottle. You can use this to clean counters, tiles, and the fridge as well. When using this mixture, spray it on the surface and let it sit for a few minutes. It helps to lift the dirt off the floor. You can then begin cleaning. You will find that the dirt lifts off with ease!

- There are times when we forget that we have a pan of food on the gas. We tend to get distracted and find that the food has burnt. All the burnt food is now stuck to the pan. It is hard to remove all that food that is stuck to the pan. However, essential oils make our life easier! You can use a few drops of lemon oil. Fill the pan with water and add a few drops of lemon oil. You will find that it is easy to remove burnt food. The lemon oil makes it easy for the water to get the burnt food and remove it. Most dishwashing soaps now use lemon oil to help clean vessels better.

- You can spray a little essential oil in your car and also in your air conditioner at home. This helps your vehicle and house smell heavenly.

Benefits of Essential Oils

This section covers the reasons about why it is best to use essential oils.

Zero Side effects:

Essential oils are all derived from plants. The extraction process has also been mentioned in the book. Since they are derived from natural sources, there are no side effects. This is why you have to choose aromatherapy over any other pharmaceutical therapies or drugs. Every human being knows that if you use any pharmaceutical drug, you may have the chance of overdose or any other side effects. But, these issues are all non – existent when it comes to essential oils. It is a known fact that regular use of essential oils will improve your health rapidly. But, you have to ensure that you do not have any allergies to essential oils. It is necessary that you choose the correct oil for your body.

Cheap and readily available:

Pharmaceutical drugs are costly! You will find that these drugs have been priced the way they are to ensure that the manufacturers and the retailers obtain a profit. They have not been priced for the general welfare of the public. When it comes to taking care of your health through pharmaceutical drugs, you will find that it is a costly affair! There is also a possibility that these drugs are not available everywhere. You can take Africa as an example! Most places all over Africa have very little exposure and have no drugs available!

When you have decided to use drugs, you will find that the quest for these drugs is more expensive when compared to any other drug. If you are looking at optimizing your costs, you will need to follow aromatherapy. Essential oils are cheap and readily available in the market. The best part is that they can be made at home! The amount that you spend on essential oils is much less when compared to any other drug that is in the market!

Market Availability:

Pharmaceutical drugs can only be purchased on the market from chemists if they have been prescribed to you by your doctor. But, essential oils are available anywhere! The supermarket or the dollar store near your house will have a broad range of essential oils available. When you go out for grocery shopping, just add a few essential oils to your list and purchase them. If you do not want to buy these essential oils, you could start planting the herbs in your backyard and extract the oils from the plants through the processes that have been mentioned below. You can prepare these oils at home yourself – the easiest techniques have been referred to in the earlier sections of this chapter. But, you will never face a difficulty when you need to purchase an essential oil.

Chronic Illness:

If you have been suffering from any chronic diseases like arthritis or sinusitis, you will be prescribed medicines that help in keeping the pain at bay. But, you will find that you need to use these drugs on a regular basis to avoid the pain. These drugs often have serious effects on your health. You can avoid these issues by using essential oils o help you reduce and relieve yourself from the pain.

Essential oils work wonderfully well when it comes to joint pain. You can massage certain oils on your joints to give you instant relief. You will also be able to get rid of a nagging cold and headache by inhaling certain essential oils. The added advantage of using essential oils is that you will be able to obtain benefits in the longer run. You would never have anticipated to getting these benefits. You will find a list of essential oils throughout the book, which can be used by you. You will also be able to identify the best oils that you will need to use for different situations.

Safe:

The drugs that have been prescribed to you by your doctor will require you to follow a diet that will ensure that the drug is effective. You will find that the drug could be fatal when you do not follow the conditions that have been mentioned to you. To make it simpler to understand, if you do not follow the rules when it comes to using the drug, there is a chance of a fatality occurring. Essential oils are not the same at all. They do not have any side effects, as mentioned above. You can consume them without worrying about any issues. But, drugs can only be consumed under a doctor's supervision. You can use essential oils without having to worry about anything!

Multiple Benefits:

The drugs that are available in pharmacies have been manufactured to cater only to a specific illness or health issue. You can never obtain multiple benefits when you are using these drugs. If you are looking at taking care of your body in a complete way, you would have to consume a lot of pills.

When it comes to essential oils, you will obtain multiple benefits! You will be able to address various issues when it comes to essential oils. For example, sandalwood oil can be used to relieve stress and also reduce your weight. You will be able to relieve yourself of headaches and also be able to control your craving for sweets. Another fact about essential oils is that

45

they can be used in different proportions to obtain multiple benefits. When you apply essential oils, you will also be able to replenish your body with the nutrients that it requires. You will be able to control any excessive damage and also prevent any damage when you use essential oils.

Detox:

Your body has a lot of toxins in it that are accumulated over the years. This is because of the food that you consume. It could also be from the pollution in your environment. You have to find a way to remove these toxins from your body. Otherwise, it can have a nasty effect on your immune system. You will also find that you have a lot of other issues if you do not remove these toxins from your body. If you use essential oils, you will be able to trick your body into removing all the toxins and restoring your immunity.

Stress Reliever:

In this fast paced world, every person feels immense amounts of stress and pressure. It has become a part of our lives. There are a lot of factors that cause your stress. But, you and every other human being, have begun to overlook these factors to carry on with life. This causes adverse effects on your health.

Stress is very good at affecting the different organs in your body. It can do this altogether too which makes it essential that you keep an eye on the amount of stress that you have. Most people have been using pills and anti–depressants to cope with stress and the anxiety. These pills have other side effects which will harm your body further leading to further stress. There are times when you may use sleeping pills because you are unable to fall asleep due to too much stress. You have to remember that stress is not a one – time thing at all! You will have to keep taking the stress pills every day if you want them to continue to work. This may also lead to addiction issues in the future.

But how will you deal with stress effectively without hurting yourself and your body? The easiest way is to use essential oils. They can be used to relax your nerves and also have a soothing effect on your body. You will have a calm mind which will help you keep stress at bay! When you use essential oils, you will be able to avoid mood swings too!

The Best Ways to Use Essential Oils

Essential oils have certain properties that are required for your body. But, you cannot use too much of this oil for your body. These oils are found in nature and may have many properties that you may not know of. Too much of this oil is corrosive to your body. This chapter will help you identify the right ways to obtain the properties of the oil through consumption and inhalation. This is what will help you function on a regular basis.

Inhaling the oil:

This is the best way to obtain the essence of the essential oil. You will be able to heighten your senses and also be able to trigger the right response from your body. This section provides you with the best methods to obtain the properties of the essential oil.

Direct Inhaling:

This is one of the simplest ways to inhale the oil! You will be able to smell the oil to gain the essence of the oil.

Diffusion:

This method is an effortless way to inhale essential oils. You will be able to inhale the oil which is in the form of the vapor. You have to find the perfect diffuser since the one that you have may affect the constituency of the oil. This diffuser will convert the essential oil into a vapor which will send it into the air.

Use a Humidifier:

This method is something that is used by people who suffer from breathing issues. You could use it when it comes to inhaling the essential oil. You will need to buy a humidifier and add water to it. Once the water has warmed enough, you will need to pour a few drops of the essential oil onto tissue paper. Place the tissue in front of the humidifier and breathe the oil in. This will help to trap the steam that is escaping.

Steam:

Take a large vessel and boil water in it. You have to add a few drops of the essential oil that you want to use to the vessel. Move your head over the vessel and cover it with a towel. Start breathing in the fumes that are being released into the water. You have to ensure that you breathe slowly to obtain the full effects of the oil.

Application of the oil on certain body parts:

You have to make sure that when you use the essential oil, you apply it and rub it onto your skin as indicated in the box. You have to make sure that you dilute the oil with vegetable oil or any other carrier oil when you are preparing it. It is best to use pure oil since that has all properties of the oil. You can apply the oil only on the body parts mentioned below.

- The forehead

- The sole of your feet

- The neck

- The temples behind the ears

- The crown of the head

- The top of your ankle

There are quite a few techniques that you can use when it comes to using essential oils on your body. The section below provides you with simple techniques that you could use.

Direct Application:

This is the best and the easiest way to administer essential oils to your body. You can take a few drops of the oil and apply it to your body for five minutes while moving your hands in a circular motion.

Massage oil:

The one way you can ensure that your body absorbs the oil is through a massage. You can use three or four drops of the essential oil and spread it all over your palms. Then you can apply the oil on the area of your skin that needs the oil. You will need to move your palms in a circular motion while exerting a certain amount of pressure. You will be able to ensure that the oil does not harm your skin in any way. You need to remember that essential oils are highly potent and will cause a bad irritation to your skin if not diluted.

If you find that you are unable to use essential oils to massage your body, you could add vegetable oil to the essential oil. This will help to balance the potency of the essential oil.

Oral Consumption:

Oral use of oils is the best way to consume the oil. But, it is dangerous since the oils do have a high potency and could cause internal damage. This may adversely affect your body. This section contains information on

54

the different ways you can consume essential oils orally.

A lot of research has been conducted which has indicated that essential oils are very effective when they have been consumed orally. This does not mean that you would sip the oil the way you would sip water. You have to ensure that the oil is in its purest form before you consume the oil. The oils are often used in dietary supplements. It is your age that determines how much of the oil needs to be diluted. You have to know what the constitution of your health is before you use the oil. You also need to read the instructions behind the product before you begin to consume it!

- You could have a capsule that is filled with the essential oil. You will have to wash it down with a lot of water since water helps in neutralizing the oil.

-   You could add a few drops of the essential oil to your milk. You should not add too much of the oil. You can add 1 or 2 drops of the oil.

-   You could add a few drops of the oil to your food when you are cooking it. This food could be bread or regular cooking.

-   You should drop the pill onto your tongue and swallow the pill immediately. You need to ensure that you are very careful when you are doing this since essential oils are highly potent. When you place the pill on your tongue, you are directly putting the oil on your tongue.

Some Precautions When Using Essential Oils

Essential oils can be potentially hazardous materials. However, when handled in the appropriate manner, the risks of using essential oils are minuscule. It is important to be aware of potential risks and follow basic guidelines when you are using essential oils. The following guide is not a complete safety reference and if you are in unsure, consult a qualified aromatherapy practitioner or your physician before continuing.

- **Essential Oils Should Never Be Used Undiluted On The Skin**: There are some instances when those who are experienced with essential oils make exceptions. However, there are many dangers to adding undiluted essential oils to the skin, and it should not be attempted without sufficient knowledge of those risks. Some instances when someone might use an essential oil undiluted, or neat, is for a bug bite, a burn, or a sting. If you are choosing to use an essential oil in this way, it is important to know that you should never use an essential oil on a child without first diluting the oil.

- **Some Oils Can Cause Sensitization Or Allergic Reactions In Some Individuals**: When you are using a new oil topically for the first time, it is important to do a skin patch test on a small area of skin before using it all over. Sensitization occurs when you become susceptible to a reaction from an essential oil that you previously didn't react to. If you find that you are suddenly reacting to an essential oil, stop using it.

To Do a Skin Patch Test: Performing a skin patch test is easy and necessary to help you determine if an essential oil is going to cause your skin to react. Keep in mind that just because you don't react to a certain essential oil, it doesn't mean that someone else may not react to it. Also, keep in mind that if you are allergic to a plant you are more than likely going to be allergic to that botanical's essential oil.

1. Place one to two drops of a diluted essential oil on the inside of your elbow. (Diluted means after the essential oil has been mixed with a carrier oil)

2. Apply a bandage or gauze to cover the area and avoid getting this area wet during the test.

3. If you feel any irritation or reaction occurring, immediately remove the bandage and wash the area with mild soap and water.

4. If there is no irritation after twenty-four hours, the diluted essential oil is safe for you to use on your skin.

- **Some Essential Oils Are Phototoxic**: Essential oils that are phototoxic can cause irritation, inflammation, redness, burning and blistering when they are exposed to UVA rays. Citrus oils as a group are considered to be phototoxic. However, there are exceptions to that rule. This is a list of citrus essential oils that are not phototoxic:

  - Lemon, steam distilled;

  - Lime, steam distilled;

  - Mandarin;

  - Sweet Orange;

  - Tangerine; and

  - furanocoumarin/bergapten free Bergamot

- **There Are Times That You Should Avoid Essential Oils**: There are some essential oils that should be avoided if you are pregnant, have asthma, epilepsy or some other health conditions. Be sure to consult your physician or a trained practitioner before using any essential oils if you have any health conditions or concerns about using essential oils.

- **Less Is More**: Essential oils are very concentrated. If a recipe calls for one to two drops of an essential oil, then that is all you are going to need to get the job done. Always make sure to use a carrier oil if you are applying essential oils to your skin.

- **Not All Essential Oils Are Suitable To Use In Aromatherapy**: There are some oils that are not meant to be used for aromatherapy. Some of these include wintergreen, rue, onion, bitter almond, and wormwood. Only use those essential oils that are recommended for use in aromatherapy. If you aren't sure, consult a trained practitioner before use.

- **Essential Oils Should Not Be Taken Internally**: Due to the high concentration of essential oils, they should not be ingested without a thorough understanding of appropriate usage and risks associated with each oil.

- **Essential Oils Are Flammable**: Keep your essential oils away from fire hazards.

Some quick pointers on using Essential Oils

Essential oils are usually highly concentrated. This is what makes them a little dangerous to use haphazardly. You have to ensure that you are able to handle yourself and the oils you use when you have decided to use them for your body. There are some rules that you will need to follow. These have been mentioned explicitly in this section of the chapter.

1. It is always good to use a drop orifice. You have to ensure that you are using the correct proportion of the oil based on what has been prescribed by your doctor or the professional whom you have been consulting. With children at home, you will need to ensure that you have an orifice that only reduces the size of the drop. This will ensure that your children or you do not consume more than is necessary. If you find that either you or your child have consumed much more than necessary, you will

need to visit the doctor immediately. But, before you go, consume a glass of milk.

2. Before you administer the oil to your children, you should meet a doctor to verify the usage of the oil for your children. It is always good to avoid any repercussions.

3. Before you begin using essential oils, you will need to ensure that they do not harm you. You have to make sure that your skin is safe from the usage of the essential oil. You should test the oil on a patch of your skin. If you find that that area has turned red or has begun to react negatively, you will need to wash the oil off immediately with water.

4. Never use oils separately. It is always good to use a blend of oils. The recipes in the book use blends of different oils. You should test these

blends too. Apply a little oil on your skin and wait for a few minutes. If you find that there is no negative response to the oil, you can continue to use it.

5. Some essential oils may affect any object and may also hurt your skin. If you find that you have used essential oils and touched your contact lenses, you may be damaging them permanently. You may also hurt your eyes in the process. Remove the lenses immediately and apply two drops of vegetable oil to your eyes.

6. You have to be very careful about your ears. Avoid applying essential oils anywhere close to your ears.

7. When you begin to use essential oils, you will find that they have a different effect on your skin when you are out in the sun.

8. If you have applied lot of cosmetics to your face, you have to refrain from using any essential oil. This is because the cosmetics will absorb the oil into your body. This oil will then be absorbed by your blood or by the fatty tissue in your body.

9. If you have any bruises or scars on your body, you have to refrain from using essential oils on those areas.

Chapter 2: Essential Oils throughout the World

Essential oils have been used by many different cultures around the world for centuries. The uses of essential oils varied between different cultures from religious practices to healing the sick. While it is difficult to pinpoint exactly when essential oils gained notoriety as being effective healing agents, the knowledge of essential oils has spread around the globe.

The earliest evidence that has been found proving human knowledge of the healing properties of the plants was located in Lascaux, which is in the Dordogne region in France. There, cave paintings were found that suggest the use of medicinal plants in everyday life that have been carbon dated as far back as 18,000 B.C.E. There has also been evidence showing that different places in the world were using essential oils even earlier. In this chapter, we are going to look at when different countries began using essential oils and how they used them.

Egypt

Recorded history has shown that Egyptians have used essential, or aromatic, oils as early as 4500 B.C.E. They have become renowned for their knowledge of cosmetology, ointments and aromatic oils. At the height of Egypt's power, only priests were allowed to use essential oils, as they were regarded as necessary to be at one with the Gods. Despite the importance that essential oils had in Egyptian society, they never distilled their own and in fact, imported oils of cypress and cedar.

China

The first uses of essential oils were recorded in Chine between 2697-2597 B.C.E during the time that Huang Ti, the legendary Yellow Emperor reigned. His famous book, "The Yellow Emperor's Book of Internal Medicine" contains uses for several aromatics, and is still used by many of the practitioners who practice eastern medicine today.

India

Ayur-Veda is a traditional Indian medicine which has a three-thousand-year history of incorporating essential oils into their healing potions. The Vedic literature contains over seven hundred substances including cinnamon, ginger, myrrh, and sandalwood as being effective for healing.

Greece

The Greeks recorded knowledge of essential oils that were adopted from the Egyptians between 400 and 500 B.C.E. Greek soldiers carried ointment of myrrh into battle with them to counter off infections.

Rome

The people of Rome were known for lavishly applying perfumed oils to their bodies, bedding, and clothing. It was customary for Romans to use oils for bathing as well as massage. These oils were what we now know as essential oil blends.

Persia

Ali-Ibn Sana, also known as Avicenna the Arab, was a well-educated physician at the age of twelve. He is known for writing books on the properties of eight hundred plants and their effects on the human body. He is also credited with being the first person to discover and record the method of distilling essential oils. His methods are still in use today.

Europe

During the time of the Crusades, the Knights and their armies were responsible for passing along knowledge of herbal medicines that they learned while they were in the Middle East. They passed this information on throughout Western Europe. Knights acquired knowledge of distillation and carried perfumed with them.

An interesting fact about essential oils in Europe is that during the Bubonic Plague of the fourteenth century, frankincense and pine were burned in the streets to ward off "evil spirits." It has been noted that there were fewer people who died of the plague in the areas where this was done.

As you can see, essential oils have been being used for many different purposes for a very long time. While there are very few scientific studies that have been done on the effects essential oils can have on the human body, there is a lot of anecdotal evidence to support the uses that essential oils have.

Chapter 3: Carrier Oils and Other Options

Carrier oils are the base oils that are used to dilute essential oils in recipes. In this chapter, we are going to look at the carrier oils that you can use with your essential oils as well as their properties. Most recipes will allow you to use your choice of carrier oil, so it is important to know what your options are and what is going to work best for you and the recipe you are using. We are going to list consistency, absorbency, aroma, shelf life and any other pertinent characteristics you should know about each carrier oil.

It is important that you use a carrier oil to dilute your essential oils as essential oils are very concentrated and can cause skin irritation if you don't. This is also true when you are using your essential oils in a distiller or to inhale. Constantly inhaling essential oils without diluting them first can lead to stripping the mucus membranes in your lungs.

As well as the carrier oils that are listed below, you can also use any lotion that you like as long as it is not made with petroleum-based oils or synthetic fragrances. The lotion is a good choice when you are looking for something with fast absorption. Because the lotion quickly absorbs, it is an excellent choice for injuries like sore muscles and joints.

Grapeseed Oil

Consistency: Liquid

Absorbency: Fairly quick, leaves a light oily sheen on the skin

Aroma: Light, slightly sweet with a hint of nuttiness

Shelf Life: Six to twelve months. Placing it in the fridge may extend the shelf life.

Best Uses: Full body massage

Other Facts: Grapeseed oil has a lower price point and is very moisturizing.

Grapeseed oil is one of the lightest carrier oils you can get on the market. As its name implies, it is extracted from the seed of grapes. The grape seeds are dried and then pressed and extracted. Grapeseed oil is cold pressed and refined to produce the light yellow-green colored oil that is popular in the cosmetic industry.

Grapeseed oil is commonly used in skincare products such as creams and lotions as well as in aromatherapy. It is popular among massage therapists because it has a smooth glide and light, satin-like finish that will not stain sheets. Grapeseed oil is easily absorbed by the skin and carries a reduce danger of allergy, making it a good choice for those with sensitive skin. Grapeseed oil also has some astringent qualities, making it a good choice if you have oily or acne prone skin.

Sweet Almond Oil

Consistency: Soft oil

Absorbency: Absorbs rapidly, leaves a slight oil on the skin

Aroma: Slightly sweet and nutty, many people feel it is odorless

Shelf Life: Six to twelve months

Best Uses: Massage oil, also ideal for individuals who spend a lot of time in the sun as it performs as a natural UV blocker

Other Facts: It is important to know that this may cause a reaction to those with allergies to nut products. Sweet almond oil is also loaded with protein making it perfect for deep tissue massages.

Sweet almond oil is obtained from the dried kernels of the almond tree. It is great for softening and soothing the skin and helps the skin balance both its loss and absorption of moisture.

Sweet almond oil is known to help relieve irritation, inflammation and itching and works well for all skin types. Sweet almond oil promotes a clear younger looker complexion and also helps to relieve muscular aches and pains when it is used as a massage oil.

Jojoba Oil

Consistency: Soft oil

Absorbency: Non-greasy absorption, very similar to the natural oils of the skin

Aroma: Slightly nutty

Shelf Life: Up to five years

Best Uses: Face wash, face mask, shampoo

Other Facts: Can be added to other carrier oils to extend their shelf life

Jojoba oil is the liquid that comes from the seed of the jojoba plant (Simmondsia Chinensis) which is a shrub that is native to southern Arizona, southern California, and northwestern Mexico. While it is referred to as oil, jojoba oil is actually a liquid plant wax.

Jojoba oil is an emollient; it is great for soothing the skin and unclogging hair follicles. It is rich in iodine which fights the harmful bacteria growth that leads to acne breakouts. Jojoba oil also contains antioxidants which soothe fine lines, wrinkles and also slow down other signs of aging.

Olive Oil

Consistency: liquid oil

Absorbency: Leaves the skin with an oily feeling

Aroma: Strong aroma

Shelf Life: eighteen months

Best Uses: rheumatic conditions, shampoos, and soaps

Other Facts: Popular and easy to find, the extra virgin varieties have more nutrients in them

Olive oil is a fruit oil that is obtained from the olive. Many people are aware of the internal health benefits, what people don't know if that olive oil also contains many benefits to the skin when used topically.

Extra virgin olive oils are the preferred variety when you are using this oil as a carrier. There are more antioxidant properties which are great for moisturizing and cleansing.

Fractionated Coconut Oil

Consistency: Liquid at room temperature

Absorbency: Absorbs well, skin will be left feeling silky

Aroma: Not noticeable

Shelf Life: Indefinite

Best Uses: Massage oil

Other Facts: This is a liquid form of coconut oil where the long-chain trans glycerides have been removed

As implied, fractionated coconut oil is a fraction of the coconut oil where almost all of the long chain triglycerides are removed leaving just the medium chain triglycerides. This makes fractionated coconut oil an absolutely saturated oil giving it a very long shelf life and increases the stability.

Fractionated coconut oil is widely used as a carrier in cosmetics, aromatherapy, and hair care. One of the disadvantages to fractionated coconut oil is that it is more expensive due to the increased amount of processing that is required. However, due to the fact it is rancid resistant, it has an indefinite shelf life and is typically worth the additional cost.

Coconut Oil

Consistency: Solid at room temperature, thick, creamy but not oily

Absorbency: readily absorbed, leaves skin feeling silky

Aroma: Very distinct coconut aroma

Shelf Life: Two to four years

Best Uses: Lotions, skin care, soap

Other Facts: Can be used to give other carrier oils a longer shelf life

Coconut oil is one of the more expensive options on the market for carrier oils. Unlike fractionated coconut oil, where the long chain triglycerides are removed, coconut oil leaves all of the triglycerides intact. This means that the shelf life is a little shorter, but you still get all of the benefits.

Since coconut oil is solid at room temperature, it is a good option if you are looking for a thick lotion. This is a great choice if you are looking for a carrier oil for an essential oil that you are going to use for skin and hair care.

Sunflower Oil

Consistency: liquid

Absorbency: Average speed absorbency, doesn't leave an oily residue

Aroma: Faint and sweet

Shelf Life: Twelve months

Best Uses: Massage and Aromatherapy

Other Facts: Bring oil to room temperature before using

Sunflower oil is obtained from the cold pressing of sunflower seeds. This method of extraction is used to ensure that all of the goodness of the sunflower seeds is retained. Sunflower oil is a light oil that doesn't leave a heavy or greasy feeling on the skin. When sunflower oil is used regularly, it provides a barrier on the skin that is resistant to infection.

Sunflower oil contains a high content of vitamin E which is an antioxidant and beneficial for healing bruises and scar tissue. The antioxidants also help prevent fine lines and wrinkles from appearing on the skin. Since sunflower oil has a very light scent, it is a good choice for essential oils that you want to be able to smell over the carrier oil.

Hazelnut Oil

Consistency: Liquid

Absorbency: Quickly absorbs and leaves a non-greasy feeling on skin

Aroma: Very mild scent

Shelf Life: Two years when refrigerated

Best Uses: Massage and aromatherapy, skin care

Other Facts: Deeply penetrating and stimulating to the circulatory system, also helps to tone and tighten the skin.

Hazelnut oil is created from both roasted as well as cold pressed hazelnuts. This oil is typically pale yellow in color. The natural fats in hazelnut oil are great for moisturizing and conditioning the skin, leaving it soft while decreasing the appearance of fine lines.

Hazelnut oil can be used in addition to sunscreen as it is able to assist in filtering the sun's rays. Hazelnut oil has a high content of catechins and tannins which make it a great choice for all skin types from the most sensitive and dry skin to the oiliest and acne ridden skin.

Wheat Germ Oil

Consistency: Liquid

Absorbency: Leaves an oily feeling on the skin, not well absorbed

Aroma: Distinct earthy aroma

Shelf Life: Two years when refrigerated

Best Uses: skin care, hair care

Other Facts: Best used in dilution with other carrier oils. Great to be added to other carrier oils to extend their shelf life naturally

Wheat germ oil is acquired from the center of the wheat berry which is called the wheat germ. The wheat germ is what supplies the plant with the nutrients to help the plan germinate and grow. Wheat germ is nutrient rich and makes a great antioxidant to help restore overall health and boost the immune system.

Wheat germ oil isn't a good choice if you have a gluten or wheat allergy or sensitivity. Wheat germ oil is high in vitamin A, E and D as well as proteins, iron, calcium, lecithin, and linoleic, palmitic, and stearic fatty acids. It is an exceptional choice for repairing dermatitis, eczema, and psoriasis.

Another option to lotion and carrier oils is a carrier butter. Butters are great when you want an essential oil to absorb slowly over a longer period.

Cocoa Butter

Consistency: Solid at room temperature

Absorbency: Average, leaves an oily barrier on the skin

Aroma: Sweet chocolate aroma

Shelf Life: Two to three years

Best Uses: Facial wrinkles, skin care, stretch marks

Other Facts: Best to use when melted and blended with other carrier oils, forms a barrier which retains the moisture in the skin while still allowing the skin to breath

Cocoa butter is a natural fat which is extracted from the cacao bean of the cacao tree. Cacao beans are found in the oval shaped pods of the cacao tree. They are harvested, fermented and dried. Once the cacao bean has been roasted and processed, it is called a cocoa bean. These cocoa beans are pressed in a hydraulic machine to produce cocoa butter from within them.

Cocoa butter is a natural moisturizer that melts just above room temperature. Because it is high in fatty acids, it is able to penetrate the skin for deep hydration. Cocoa butter contains antioxidants which give it antiaging properties, as well as the ability to help reduce the appearance of stretch marks, age spots and scars.

Shea Butter

Consistency: Soft oil, semi-solid

Absorbency: Average, leaves a waxy feeling on the skin

Aroma: Distinct nutty odor

Shelf Life: One to two years

Best Uses: Lip balm, dry skin, stretch marks

Other Facts: Effective to use "as is" or in a compound of carriers

Shea butter comes from the seeds of the fruit of the Shea or Karite tree. It is naturally rich in vitamins A, E and F. Shea butter offers low levels of skin protection from UV rays, around an SPF of six. Shea butter is high in fatty acids and other nutrients which enable it to help the production of collagen.

Shea butter is nourishing and moisturizing for the skin and can help both dry and oily skin. Raw, unrefined Shea butter is the best choice when you are selecting a Shea butter because the refining process removes some of the beneficial properties of the oil. When you purchase unrefined oil, it is helpful to melt the oil and pour it through a cheesecloth to remove any of the trace particles of nut that might remain.

Some Safety Issues to Consider When Using Carriers

It is important to consider the shelf life of your carriers when you are pre-mixing your blends. While essential oils are safe for up to eight years, most carriers are only suitable for six to twelve months. Making smaller batches will ensure you can get through the entire batch before the carrier goes rancid. Toss out any carrier oils that have become cloudy have a foul odor or go rancid.

It is recommended to avoid using soy oils, canola oils and most other vegetable oils as carrier oils. Also, avoid using any oils that are refined, processed or non-organic. Raw and organic oils are the best to use as carrier oils.

It is also not recommended to use water as a carrier as water does not mix well with essential oils. Although some bath products work best when mixed with water, if you are applying the product directly to the skin, you may not get an even amount of the essential oil when mixing with water.

Take into consideration any allergies or sensitivities you might have to a carrier oil when you are making your selection. If you are trying a carrier oil for the first time, it is a good idea to do a skin patch test for an allergy to ensure that you are able to use it. This is especially important if you are also using an essential oil for the first time, so that if you have a reaction to the mixture you are able to pinpoint what you reacted to.

Chapter 4: Best Essential Oils for Anti-Aging

Essential oils are a great choice when you are looking for an anti-aging treatment that is going to really work, isn't going to cost a lot of money and smells amazing. When you are purchasing over the counter anti-aging treatments, you are going to spend a lot more money, and these treatments often have ingredients in them that are unfamiliar.

When you are using essential oils on your face, and especially around your eyes, you need to be aware that the essential oil might react with the skin. Essential oils are a natural and healthy approach to countering the aging of our skin. In addition to all of the anti-aging benefits, these oils are also going to keep your skin smelling good throughout the day.

There are many things that can lead to premature aging of our skin. Smoking, alcohol use, sun exposure and a poor diet all contribute to wrinkles, age spots, and tired and dull looking skin. Here we are going to cover some of the best essential oils for aging skin. Once we are familiar with the options of essential oils, we are going to look at some recipes that they can be used in.

Geranium Essential Oil: This essential oil has a flowery scent. It has a natural astringent effect that tightens skin. The tightening of the skin reduces large pores which tones and firms aging skin. Geranium essential oil also promotes cell renewal and blood circulation. This essential oil also steers away free radicals that steal oxygen and cause the degeneration of healthy skin cells.

Botanical Name – Pelargonium Graveolens or Pelargonium Asperum

Color – Ranges in color from clear to amber

Perfumery Note – Middle

Sandalwood Essential Oil: This essential oil is a great option to protect skin cells from UV radiation and sun damage. The natural astringent properties help to tighten, firm and improve the tone of your skin. Sandalwood Essential Oil contains skin regenerative properties that are great for improving circulation and promoting smoother looking skin.

Botanical Name – Santalum Album

Color – Clear with a yellow tinge

Perfumery Note – Base

Frankincense Essential Oil: This essential oil is perhaps one of the best for aging skin. It minimizes the appearance of scars, stretch marks, and age spots. Frankincense essential oil balances the skin's pH and also helps to tighten and firm sagging skin.

Botanical Name – Boswellia Carterii

Color – Light yellow

Perfumery Note – Base

Rose Essential Oil: This essential oil helps with the elasticity of the skin by preventing the breakdown of collagen and delaying wrinkles. Rose essential oil has a flowery, romantic scent and is great for improving circulation.

Botanical Name – Rosa Damascena

Color – Deep red

Perfumery Note – Middle

Myrrh Essential Oil: This essential oil is an excellent choice to smooth out aging skin and prevent wrinkles under the eyes from forming. Myrrh essential oil helps by improving the flow of oxygen throughout the skin.

Botanical Name – Commiphora Myrrha

Color – Golden yellow to brown

Perfumery Note – Base

Lavender Essential Oil: This essential oil contains anti-inflammatory, anti-aging, antifungal and antimicrobial properties. Lavender essential oil is great for delaying fine line wrinkles, age spots, and sun spots thanks to its regenerative properties.

Botanical Name – Lavandula Angustifolia or Lavandula Officianalis

Color – Clear with a tinge of yellow

Perfumery Note – Top to middle

Carrot Seed Essential Oil: This is an essential oil that is rich in vitamins, minerals, and antioxidants that help to protect skin from sun damage as well as delay signs of aging. Carrot seed essential oil is great for tightening the skin and promoting cell regeneration.

Botanical Name – Daucus Carota

Color – Golden yellow

Perfumery Note – Middle

Chapter 5: Essential Oil Recipes for Anti-Aging

Now that we have an understanding of essential oils that are great for reversing the aging of our skin, we are going to take a look at some recipes you can use. Here are six great recipes to undo the damage that time has done to your skin.

Face Oil: This is a great oil to use as part of your skin care routine to maintain smooth, youthful looking skin.

In an amber glass bottle with a dropper, mix:

- Five (5) drops of sandalwood essential oil

- Three (3) drops of geranium essential oil

- Two (2) tablespoons of sweet almond oil

Anti-Wrinkle Treatment: Apply this oil to your face twice a day for ten days. Continue using once every two days to stimulate the production of collagen and delay the formation of under eye wrinkles.

In a glass dropper bottle mix:

- Three (3) drops of frankincense essential oil

- Four (4) drops of carrot seed essential oil

- Seven (7) tablespoons of jojoba oil

Massage Oil to Delay Aging: Massage this oil into your face and neck daily to prevent signs of premature aging and to help promote proper blood circulation.

In a dark glass bottle mix:

- Ten (10) drops of lavender essential oil

- Two (2) Ounces of liquid coconut oil

Under Eye Healing Blend: Apply this healing blend by dotting it under the eyes and on the face. Massage gently until the skin has soaked it up.

In a small cobalt blue glass dropper bottle mix:

- Seven to Ten (7-10) of myrrh essential oil

- Two (2) tablespoons of jojoba oil

Anti-Aging Serum: Apply this anti-aging serum to your face every evening right before bed to bring back your youthful and glowing skin.

In a glass dropper bottle mix:

- Five to seven (5-7) drops of geranium essential oil

- Three to five (3-5) drops of lemon essential oil

- Half (1/2) of a cup of sweet almond oil

Moisturizing Cream: This moisturizing cream will rejuvenate and provide deep hydration for aging skin all over the body. Just apply a pea sized amount once a day.

In a small jar mix:

- Four (4) drops of rose essential oil

- Two (2) tablespoons of Shea butter

Chapter 6: Best Essential Oils for Face Care

In this chapter, we are going to have a look at some of the best essential oils to use on your face to treat acne, scars, as well as blackheads. We are also going to describe the best essential oils for face washes for oily, dry, normal and combination skin types.

Tea Tree Essential Oil: This essential oil is anti-bacterial which helps to ward off the bacteria that cause acne. Tea tree essential oil also regulates oil production which contributes to decrease the sensitivity of the skin and the number of breakouts that occur.

Botanical Name – Melaleuca Alternifolia

Color – Clear with a yellow tinge

Perfumery Note – Middle

Lemongrass Essential Oil: This essential oil contains invigorating and antiseptic properties. Lemongrass Essential Oil is an excellent choice in facial toners as it contains astringent properties that help fight greasy skin and acne.

Botanical Name – Cymbopogon Citratus or Cymbopogon Flecuosus

Color – Pale yellow to vivid yellow

Perfumery Note – Top

Ylang-ylang Essential Oil: This is a great essential oil for every skin type to help control oil production and minimize breakouts. Ylang-ylang essential oil also aids in the regeneration of skin cells and improves the elasticity of the skin.

Botanical Name – Cananga Odorata Var Genuina

Color – Clear with a yellow tinge

Perfumery Note – Middle to base

Neroli Essential Oil: This is an excellent essential oil choice for skin that is oily or sensitive. Neroli essential oil contains a naturally occurring chemical called citral which regenerates cells. It also contains antiseptic properties which contribute to balancing oil production and shrinking the appearance of pores while keeping the skin moisturized.

Botanical Name – Citrus Aurantium

Color – Orange to brown

Perfumery Note – Middle

Patchouli Essential Oil: This is a great essential oil for acne due to its antiseptic, antifungal and antibacterial properties. Patchouli essential oil also promotes the growth of new cell growth and aids in the smoothing of fine lines.

Botanical Name – Pogostemon Cablin

Color – Deep golden brown

Perfumery Note – Base

Roman Chamomile Essential Oil: This essential oil is an excellent choice for all skin types that are looking for a gentle essential oil. Roman chamomile essential oil offers a soft scent as well as being gentle on the skin.

Botanical Name – Anthemis Nobilis or Chamaemelum Nobile

Color – Gray to a very pale blue

Perfumery Note –Middle

Myrtle Essential Oil: This is an essential oil effective in the treatment and prevention of acne and pimples.

Botanical Name – Myrtus Communis

Color – Pale Yellow

Perfumery Note – Top to middle

Some of the other essential oils that are perfect for face care were already covered in Chapter 3. These essential oils include lavender, myrrh, geranium and carrot seed essential oils.

Chapter 7: Essential Oil Recipes for Face Care

There are an incredible number of essential oils that you can choose from to gain different health benefits. Below you will find some recipes for face care including various options for face cleansers and treatments for pimples, blemishes, and acne. Keep in mind that you can replace the carrier oils if you find that the one that is in the recipe doesn't work for you or your skin. When you replace the carrier oils, replace them with one that is the same consistency to achieve a similar product.

Some of these recipes are going to call for rose water. This is water that has been scented with rose petals and can be replaced with filtered or distilled water if you prefer. A note when you are purchasing rose water, ensure that you are buying pure rose water and not one that is loaded with preservatives or artificial rose scent as these won't have the same benefits to your skin.

Peppermint Toner: Use this toner after washing your face in the morning and the evening. You can apply this toner by lightly misting your face with a spray bottle, or it can be used with a cotton ball. Store this toner in the refrigerator.

In a glass spray bottle or any glass bottle, mix:

- Twenty to fifty (20-50) drops of peppermint essential oil

- Three-quarters (3/4) of a cup of filtered water

- One-quarter (1/4) cup of apple cider vinegar

116

Lemon Toner: This toner is meant for those who have large pores. This toner is intended to be used once a day in the morning. Apply this toner by either lightly misting your face with a spray bottle or with a cotton ball.

In a glass spray bottle or any glass bottle, mix:

- One to two (1-2) drops of lemon essential oil

- One and a half (1 ½) cups of distilled water

- One-half (1/2) teaspoon of lemon juice

Make-Up Remover: This recipe is perfect for removing any makeup that you wear including those water proof ones that never want to leave your skin. Simply dip a cotton ball or soft cloth into the make-up remover and apply to your face.

In a small jar, mix:

- One (1) drop of Roman chamomile essential oil

- Two (2) tablespoons of jojoba oil

- One-half (1/2) cup of mild castile soap

- One-half (1/2) cup filtered water

Acne Treatment Gel: This gel is great for spot treating pimples and acne. Just apply the gel at night to the problems areas on your face and you will notice an improvement by morning.

In a small jar, mix:

- Four (4) drops of geranium essential oil

- Five (5) teaspoons of shea butter

Facial Cleanser for Normal Skin: This face wash is gentle and efficient at cleansing and moisturizing any skin type, but it is most beneficial for those with normal skin types. To use this cleanser, dampen your face with warm water. Gently massage the face cleanser into your skin rinse and pat dry. Let cure for 24 hours after making.

In a dark glass bottle, mix:

- Eight (8) drops of lavender essential oil

- One (1) drop of geranium essential oil

- One (1) drop of Ylang-ylang essential oil

- Two-thirds (2/3) cup of rose water

- One (1) tablespoon of Shea butter

Facial Cleanser for Combination Skin: This facial cleanser is perfect for combination skin as it is moisturizing, cleansing and balancing for your skin while still being incredibly gentle. To use this cleanser, dampen your face with warm water. Gently massage the face cleanser into your skin, rinse and pat dry. Let cure for 24 hours after making.

In a dark glass bottle, mix:

- Four (4) drops of lavender essential oil

- Three (3) drops of lemongrass essential oil

- Two (2) drops of geranium essential oil

- One (1) drop of ylang-ylang essential oil

- One-half (1/2) cup of rose water

- Two (2) tablespoons of Shea butter

- Two (2) tablespoons of aloe vera gel

Facial Cleanser for Dry Skin: This cleanser is ideal for dry skin. This combines deep cleaning with intense moisture to help prevent rough scaly patches from forming. Only use this facial cleanser once a day before bedtime to prevent your skin from drying out from over washing.

In a dark glass bottle, mix:

- Four (4) drops roman chamomile essential oil

- Four (4) drops geranium essential oil

- Six (6) drops orange essential oil

- Four (4) tablespoons sunflower seed oil

Facial Cleanser for Sensitive Skin: This cleanser is an excellent choice for those with sensitive skin. Made with an olive oil base, this cleanser promotes smooth, healthy skin that will heal and cleanse your face without damaging it. To use this face cleanser, pour a small amount into your hand and massage it into your face, focusing on any area that is irritated. Once your skin is saturated in the cleanser, take a hot cloth and let it sit on your face until it cools. This will remove the olive oil as well as all the dirt. After the cloth has cooled, rinse the cloth and gently wipe the oil away. Do this three to four times daily.

In a dark glass bottle, mix:

- Twelve (12) drops lavender essential oil

- Two (2) drops neroli essential oil

- One (1) drop roman chamomile essential oil

- One-half (1/2) cup extra virgin olive oil

Facial Cleanser for Acne and Oily Skin: This cleanser is ideal for oily and acne ridden skin. It will cleanse your face and prevent your face from overproducing oils which can lead to acne.

In a dark glass bottle, mix:

- Six (6) drops lavender essential oil

- Six (6) drops tea tree essential oil

- Two (2) drop lemongrass essential oil

- Four (4) tablespoons of grapeseed oil

Clarifying face exfoliant: Do you find that your skin has started to look dull? This exfoliant helps in clearing and brightening your skin. You will find that you can treat any new acne that has popped on your skin. You will also find that you can clear any old blemishes that you may have on your skin.

Ingredients:

- Baking Soda
- Fresh Lime Juice
- Tea Tree Oil

Method:

- Take a small bowl.

- Mix one tablespoon of Lime juice.

- Add two tablespoons of baking soda to the bowl.

- Mix well. Ensure that there are no lumps.

- Now add three drops of tea tree oil and mix.

- You have to remember that Lime juice is acidic and can irritate your skin.

- You have to ensure that you dilute the mixture of the oil with water if you have dry skin.

- Now mix these ingredients into a paste. Make sure that it is smooth and has all the right measurements.

- Apply the paste onto your face using your fingertips. You will need to move your fingers in circles to ensure that you move your fingertips in the clockwise direction.

- Let the paste stay on your face for a few minutes.

- Wash your face with warm water and pat dry. As an alternative, you could use cotton to wipe off the paste and then wash your face with warm water.

Note: If you exfoliate too much, you will start causing a lot of irritation to your skin. You will find that you have begun having a lot of acne. It is best to exfoliate your skin once a week! If you have oily skin, you could exfoliate twice.

How the exfoliant works:

You may have begun to wonder how this is the best exfoliant for your skin. This section will clear your doubts regarding the same.

The baking soda in your exfoliant is the best exfoliant ever! I cannot repeat myself enough. Baking soda is fine grained is non – abrasive when compared with any other exfoliant. It acts like a polish and helps in removing all the dead skin cells. This helps in creating or giving you a smooth complexion without any irritations or rashes on your skin. This helps in clearing all the blocked pores which in turn helps in keeping the acne away.

When you apply the lime juice on your skin, you will gain multiple benefits. Lime juice is antibacterial and provides your skin with the natural treatment that it needs against acne. It also helps in removing any blemishes that you may have on your skin. This will leave you with the confidence that you will never have another breakout of acne at that particular spot.

Lime juice also contains citric acid which helps in exfoliating the skin without causing it any harm. Lime juice also has Vitamin C which helps in clearing away the dark spots and lightening the tone of your skin. It has also been proven that Vitamin C helps in reducing wrinkles by increasing the production of collagen. Lime juice has another great property which makes it perfect to use on skin. It helps in balancing the pH of your skin! This helps in reducing any form of acne on your skin!

Tea tree oil in your exfoliant has a powerful antibacterial property that helps it keep your skin clean and away from the bacteria causing the acne.

Face blend for dry skin: Your skin may be dehydrated. You may find that there are different patches on your skin due to this. You can use this to ensure that your skin color has blended well together.

Ingredients:

- 4 drops Neroli oil

- 2 drops Roman Chamomile Oil

- 2 Tbsp. Sweet Almond Oil

Method:

- Take a bottle and add the oils.

- The almond oil makes sure that it protects your skin from coming to any harm due to the usage of the oils.

- Leave the oil in the bottle for two days. This is to ensure that the carrier oils have blended with each other.

- Once the oils have blended, you can use the mixture on your skin. You can use as much as you need. Ensure that you only use it once you have cleansed and toned your skin.

Face blend for normal skin:

Ingredients:

- 2 drops Geranium oil

- 4 drops Lavender oil

- 2 Tbsp. Sweet Almond oil

Method:

- Take a glass bottle.

- Add essential oils in the order mentioned above.

- When you have cleansed and toned your face, you should apply a few drops of the blend on your skin.

<u>Foaming face wash:</u> Most of us use a face wash every morning to scrub their face clean of the previous night's sleep. But, this face wash is loaded with chemicals that may lead to a lot of acne in the future. Instead, you could switch to products that have very little chemicals and are more natural. This will help in gaining a clear skin. You will find that you have great and gentle skin once you start using the foaming face wash that has been mentioned below.

Ingredients:

- One cup filtered water (boil this to room temperature)

- 7 Tsp. Jojoba oil. You could use any other facial oil if you prefer that. It is best to use jojoba oil since that oil does not clog pores that are it has a low comedogenic rating. You could also use sunflower oil since it has a low comedogenic rating too.

- 20 drops of lemon essential oil. This is a natural antibacterial oil that will help in keeping your safe clean. It also helps in fighting the bacteria that cause the acne.

- ½ cup liquid castile soap. This is the soap that is highly concentrated in the plant oils.

- 4 Tbsp. Raw honey. This is a great antibacterial. This helps in washing away all the bacteria that is capable of causing acne. It

133

also helps in keeping your skin calm and glowing. You will find that your skin is now the color of honey!

- 2 Tbsp. Tea tree oil. This oil is brilliant antibacterial oil. It is also antifungal and antimicrobial. It jells in clearing your skin of all the bacteria and also helps in keeping your skin safe after the wash.

Method:

- Take a small mixing bowl.

- Add the hot water to the bowl.

- Now add the liquid castile soap. Then follow with the remaining ingredients. Never add the soap before the water. If you do that you will only end up with a sticky paste!

- You will need to stir the mixture well to ensure that it holds together.

- Your mixture will need to look cloudy. Only then will you be able to state that the mixture is done.

- You can put the mixture in a soap dispenser and start using it!

You do not have to use too much of the soap. It is always good to only use one or two pumps. This is because castile soap is highly concentrated, and too much of anything is bad for you! It is always good to use the soap twice – once in the morning and once before you go to bed. There may be a few changes in the soap after a few days. You will have to keep an eye on the soap. When you see some unfavorable content in your soap, you can throw the soap out. Always shake the soap before you use it since this will help in mixing the content.

Note: The ingredients mentioned above may work on all skins. But, it is always good to experiment. You can change the amount of the ingredients used if you find that the amount is too much. If you have dry skin, you will have to add more oil to keep the freshness. You have to ensure that you give this a shot since you will be able to know what works best for your skin.

Chapter 8: Best Essential Oils for Hair Care

Now that you know how essential oils can help to reverse premature aging as well as how to use essential oils in general face care, we are going to have a look at what essential oils are great to use for hair care. Regardless of your hair type, there is an essential oil that is right for you.

Cedar wood Essential Oil: This essential oil is optimal for reducing dry, flaky skin on the scalp. It is also known to be helpful in aiding the growth of hair and thickening hair as well.

Botanical Name – Cadres Atlantic

Color – Light Golden Yellow

Perfumery Note - Base

Rosemary Essential Oil: If you find that you are always losing hair after you shampoo your hair, this essential oil is exactly what you are looking for. Rosemary essential oil is great for reducing hair loss, slowing down the graying process, and treating dandruff.

Botanical Name – Rosmarinus Officinalis

Color – Clear

Perfumery Note – Middle

Cypress Essential Oil: This essential oil is well known for treating alopecia areata, which is a condition that results in the loss of hair. Cypress essential oil is also great for helping to clear an oily scalp.

Botanical Name – Cupressus Sempervirens

Color – Pale yellow

Perfumery Note – Medium

<u>Clary Sage Essential Oil</u>: This essential oil is an excellent choice to help if you suffer from an inflamed, greasy or otherwise problematic scalp. Clary Sage essential oil contributes to the optimization of your scalps pH value.

Botanical Name – Salvia Sclarea

Color – Light golden yellow

Perfumery Note – Middle

Bergamot Essential Oil: This essential oil contributes to the growth of hair as well as soothing the scalp, protecting the hair and giving it a great shine.

Botanical Name – Citrus Bergamia

Color – Green to golden yellow

Perfumery Note – Top

Lemon Essential Oil: This essential oil is a great choice if you deal with dandruff or have dry curly hair. Lemon essential oil is known to stimulate the oil glands and leads to the production of more oil. This leads to hair that is shinier, healthier and stronger.

Botanical Name – Citrus Limon

Color – Pale yellow to deep yellow

Perfumery Note - Top

Some other oils that are also great for the hair that we have already discussed include carrot seed essential oil, lavender essential oil, geranium essential oil, patchouli essential oil as well as many others.

Chapter 9: Essential Oil Recipes For Hair Care

Hair care is an important aspect of self-care for many people. As people age, they start to worry about their hair drying out, thinning, graying and even becoming oily. Just like our faces, everyone's hair is a little different. Below are some great recipes to use essential oils in your hair's routine to keep it shiny, healthy and gorgeous.

<u>Dry Scalp Soak</u>: This soak is great if you have a scalp that is always itchy. Rub the soak into your scalp for two to three minutes and then allow it to sit for sixty to ninety minutes. Rinse in warm water.

In a glass container, mix:

- Six (6) drops of cedar wood essential oil

- Four (4) drops of lavender essential oil

- Two (2) drops of geranium essential oil

- Two (2) drops of patchouli essential oil

- Two-thirds (2/3) of a cup of jojoba oil

<u>Oily Scalp Soak</u>: This soak is deeply cleansing if your hair often produces too much oil. Just massage into your scalp for two to three minutes and allow it to soak in for sixty to ninety minutes. Rinse in warm water.

In a glass container, mix:

- Six (6) drops of peppermint essential oil

- Four (4) drops of lemon essential oil

- Two (2) drops of lavender essential oil

- One-half (1/2) of a cup of olive oil

Hair Loss Prevention Soak: This soak is great for coercing the hair follicles and preventing your hair from falling out during washing and brushing. Massage the oil into your scalp and allow it to soak overnight while you are sleeping.

In a glass container, mix:

- Four (4) drops of rosemary essential oil

- Four (4) drops of thyme essential oil

- Four (4) drops of lavender essential oil

- Four (4) drops of cedar wood essential oil

- Two (2) drops of frankincense essential oil

- Two (2) teaspoons of coconut oil

Dandruff Treatment: This dandruff treatment is a great and fast treatment for those who are suffering from dandruff. Simply massage into your scalp for two to three minutes and rinse out afterward.

In a glass container, mix:

- Five (5) drops of lemon essential oil

- Two (2) drops lavender essential oil

- Two (2) drops peppermint essential oil

- One (1) drop rosemary essential oil

- One (1) teaspoon jojoba oil

<u>Shampoo for Dry Hair</u>: This shampoo is deeply moisturizing to help bring some life back into your dry hair. Simply use this like regular shampoo.

In a glass container, mix:

- Four (4) drops of ylang-ylang essential oil

- Four (4) drops of geranium essential oil

- Ten (10) drops of sandalwood essential oil

- Two (2) drops of lemon essential oil

- One-quarter (1/4) cup of castile soap

- One-quarter (1/4) cup of olive oil

<u>Shampoo for Thin Hair</u>: This shampoo is great for adding body to your hair, especially if you naturally have thin, baby like hair. Use like regular shampoo.

In a glass container, mix:

- Five (5) drops of ylang-ylang essential oil

- Five (5) drops of cedar wood essential oil

- Five (5) drops of rosemary essential oil

- Five (5) drops of lavender essential oil

- One-quarter (1/4) cup of castile soap

- One-quarter (1/4) cup of jojoba oil

Shampoo for Oily Scalp: This shampoo is an invigorating way to help your scalp eliminate the added oils that it is producing. Simply use this like any shampoo.

In a glass container, mix:

- Sixteen (16) drops of rosemary essential oil

- Two (2) drops of peppermint essential oil

- One-half (1/2) cup castile soap

- One-half (1/2) cup distilled or filtered water

De tangle conditioning spray: This spray is every person's best friend. When you have long hair, you find that your hair tangles a lot in the wind and the rain. To be very honest, your hair tangles in any weather or condition!

If your hair is dry, you will need to spray enough to dampen your hair. Run your comb or your brush through your hair. This spray will help in detangling and conditioning your hair. You will not find any residue on your hair either. It has been found that this spray removed frizziness too! You could also use the spray right after you wash your hair.

Ingredients:

- 2 cups Distilled water

- 2 tsp. carrot seed oil (cold pressed)

- 1 Tsp. Lavender oil

- 1 Tsp. Rosemary oil

- 1 Tbsp. solubiliser

Method:

- Take a spray bottle

- Add the distilled water to the bottle.

- Add the solubilizer and shake the spray bottle well.

- Add the oils in the order mentioned above and shake the oils well.

- You have to leave the bottle for a day to ensure that the oils have blended well.

- Apply on wet or dry hair.

Hair Loss: This is a problem that most human beings have started to face. It is most often due to extreme amounts of stress and pressure. The recipe mentioned below helps in reducing the loss of hair.

Ingredients:

- 2 Tsp. Carrot seed oil

- ½ Tsp. Clary sage oil

- 2 Tbsp. Jojoba oil

- 1 Tsp. Lavender oil

- 1 Tsp. Roman chamomile oil

- ½ Tsp. Rosemary oil

- 2 Tbsp. Sweet almond oil

Method:

- Take a clean bottle.

- Add the oils in the order mentioned above.

- Shake the bottle well.

- Heat the oil a little before you use it.

- Apply a few drops of the oil before you sleep onto your scalp.

- You have to leave it overnight to ensure that it is absorbed. You can wash it off the following morning.

- You will need to apply this oil quite a few times a week initially. But, once your hair stops falling, you could use the oil a little less frequently.

Chapter 10: Best Essential Oils for General Body Care

The term body care may seem a little broad. In this chapter, we are going to look at essential oils that are great for muscle care, your digestive tract, your teeth and even healing cuts and bruises.

<u>Clove Essential Oil</u>: This essential oil is known for the antiviral and antimicrobial properties it contains which is why the most common use is for dental care. Clove essential oil is also a great choice for supporting a healthy digestive system and increasing circulation.

Botanical Name – Eugenia Caryophyllata

Color – Golden yellow to brown

Perfumery Note – Middle

Black Pepper Essential Oil: This essential oil is highly warming and known for improving circulation. Black pepper essential oil is a great choice to help with the relief of arthritis, sore muscles, pre-exercise pain prevention and even to reduce stiffness.

Botanical Name – Piper Nigrum

Color – Clear

Perfumery Note – Middle

Ginger Essential Oil: This essential oil is great for easing muscle spasms and soothing painful joints. Ginger essential oil combines warming action with analgesic properties to support muscles.

Botanical Name – Zingiber Officinale

Color – Light Yellow

Perfumery Note – Middle to base

Eucalyptus Essential Oil: This essential oil contains analgesics as well as anti-inflammatory properties to relieve sore joints and muscles.

Botanical Name – Eucalyptus Globulus

Color – Clear

Perfumery Note – Top

Marjoram Essential Oil: This essential oil is beneficial for high blood pressure, arthritis, circulation and even indigestion. It contains soothing, warming and antispasmodic properties making it a great choice for many reasons.

Botanical Name – Origanum Majorana

Color – Clear with a tinge of yellow

Perfumery Note – Middle

Tarragon Essential Oil: This essential oil possesses properties that make it an anti-rheumatic. It is also a great oil because of its digestive and circulatory properties.

Botanical Name – Artemisia Dracunculus

Color – Clear to pale yellow

Perfumery Note – Middle

Fennel Essential Oil: This essential oil is an antiseptic essential oil that also contains expectorant, laxative and diuretic properties that all contribute to a healthy digestive system.

Botanical Name – Foeniculum Vulgare

Color – Clear with a faint yellow tinge

Perfumery Note – Top to middle

Helichrysum Essential Oil: This essential oil can safely be applied on wounds, cuts, pricks and other open sores that have the potential to become infected. Helichrysum is also a coagulant which means that it will also help stop the bleeding. This essential oil can be applied directly to a cut without needing to be added to any carrier oil. It is one of just a few oils that can do this.

Botanical Name – Helichrysum Angustifolia

Color – Light yellow

Perfumery Note – Base

There are also many other essential oils that we have already covered that you will see in the recipes in the next chapter. This is because there are many essential oils that are great for many purposes. Choosing to use these multipurpose oils is a great idea as you will need to immediately invest in less of a variety of essential oils as you begin your journey into essential oils.

You will also find a more comprehensive list of essential oils in chapter eleven.

Chapter 11: Essential Oil Recipes for General Body Care

Many people would never consider using essential oils to treat cuts, bruises, and sore muscles. Many of these recipes are cheaper and better for you than the things you are going to find on the counters of the store. In this chapter, you will find recipes for these things plus toothpaste and to help with your digestive tract.

Simple Bruise Oil: This oil will help reduce the appearance of bruising by helping to promote circulation and healing the damaged tissue. Gently massage this oil directly onto your bruise.

In a glass container, mix:

- Two (2) drops of geranium essential oil

- Two (2) drops of rosemary essential oil

- One (1) drop of lavender essential oil

- One (1) teaspoon of jojoba oil

Muscle Fatigue Massage Oil: The oils in this recipe are great for reenergizing tired muscles and helping them recover from a hard workout. The best way to use this is to massage it into your tired muscles after a warm bath or shower.

In a glass container, mix:

- Ten (10) drops of rosemary essential oil

- Ten (10) drops of eucalyptus essential oil

- Five (5) drops of cypress essential oil

- Five (5) drops of thyme essential oil

- Two (2) tablespoons of sweet almond oil

Muscle Relief Massage Oil: The oils that are used in this recipe are great for aiding in relieving sore and tired muscles, especially for those who are suffering from arthritis or poor circulation. The best way to use this is to massage it into your tired muscles after a warm bath or shower.

In a glass container, mix:

- Fifteen (15) drops of juniper essential oil

- Fifteen (15) drops of marjoram essential oil

- Ten (10) drops of rosemary essential oil

- Five (5) drops of black pepper essential oil

- Three (3) tablespoons of grapeseed oil

<u>Massage Oil For Over Exerted Muscles</u>: This blend of massage oil is great if you have overused your muscles and are looking for a way to help them relax.

The best way to use this is to massage it into your tired muscles after a warm bath or shower.

In a glass container, mix:

- Five (5) drops of eucalyptus essential oil

- Five (5) drops of ginger essential oil

- Five (5) drops of peppermint essential oil

- One (1) tablespoon of sweet almond oil

Massage Oil For Muscle Cramps: This is great massage oil if you are suffering from any muscle cramping. The best way to use this is to massage it into your tired muscles after a warm bath or shower.

In a glass container, mix:

- Five (5) drops of marjoram essential oil

- Five (5) drops of rosemary essential oil

- Five (5) drops of lavender essential oil

- Three (3) drops of black pepper essential oil

- Five (5) teaspoons of coconut oil

Sore Muscle Soak: This muscle soak is a great addition to your warm bath when you are sore and are looking for the best way to relax your tired muscles. Follow this up with one of the massage oils above and you will be on the road to healthier muscles before you know it.

Add the following essential oils to your warm bath

- Three (3) drops of marjoram essential oil

- Two (2) drops of lemon essential oil

Massage Oil For Rheumatism: This massage oil is a great blend for those who are suffering from rheumatoid arthritis and are looking for a safe and effective way to soothe their joints. The best way to use this is to massage it into your joints after a warm bath or shower.

In a glass container, mix:

- Four (4) drops of cypress essential oil

- Three (3) drops of rosemary essential oil

- Two (2) drops of juniper essential oil

- Two (2) drops of roman chamomile essential oil

- Four (4) teaspoons of sweet almond oil

<u>Before Workout Massage Oil</u>: This is a great massage oil to rub into your muscles before you work out to help prevent any overexertion of your muscles.

It will help your muscles remain supple and warm them up.

In a glass container, mix:

- Ten (10) drops of rosemary essential oil

- Ten (10) drops of pine essential oil

- Five (5) drops of grapefruit essential oil

- Five (5) drops of black pepper essential oil

- Two (2) ounces of coconut oil

Toothpaste: This toothpaste is a better option than many of the over the counter options that are available. Since it is an all-natural product, there are no risks in children accidently swallowing the toothpaste, and it is also great for freshening your breath. To avoid contamination, use a spoon or a disposable wooden scoop to get the paste out if you use a jar.

In a small glass jar or a squeeze container, mix:

- Two (2) drops of peppermint essential oil

- Two (2) drops of clove essential oil

- Two (2) drops of orange essential oil

- One to two (1-2) teaspoons of sea salt

- One-quarter (1/4) cup of baking soda

- One-quarter (1/4) cup of coconut oil

Massage Oil To Aid Digestion: To support normal digestion, it is important to massage your digestion oil on your stomach in the proper manner. Looking down at your belly button, you want to begin just below the belly button and gently massage the oils in the gentle circular motion to the right (clockwise)

In a glass container, mix:

- Five (5) drops of ginger essential oil

- Five (5) drops of peppermint essential oil

- Five (5) drops of cardamom essential oil

- Five (5) drops of fennel essential oil

- One (1) tablespoon of olive oil

Chapter 12: Best Essential Oils for Stress Relief

There has been a lot of research that has been conducted on stress. It has been found that close to 90 percent of people approach a doctor because they have been suffering from chronic headaches. They have been diagnosed with chronic stress. There are quite a few illnesses that could be caused due to stress. Heart disease is the most common of those illnesses! There is a possibility of death when you are under too much pressure. There is another fact that your body may perceive a lot of stress which in reality may or may not exist. It is because of this that you find yourself feeling stressed. You will find that when your brain has not identified the real cause of stress, it will start worrying. This is when you find yourself under immense stress.

A person who is suffering from chronic stress can be treated with essential oils. This is the most common treatment that is used all over the world. The oils contain components that help in producing a sense of calm and relief throughout the body. Essential oils can either produce a sense of calm or act as stimulants depending on what the person who it is administered on is feeling. For instance, if oil is administered by an individual who is suffering from chronic stress, it could be inducing a calming effect on him. However, if it is administered by an individual who is feeling very low, the oil may leave the person with the feeling of ecstatic joy! These oils are called adaptogens in aromatherapy. They have been christened with this name since they adapt to what the individual needs.

The following section below gives you the list of essential oils that can be used to release stress. They are the most common ones used when compared to the other oils that are known.

Cedarwood: Cedarwood is a plant that has been known all over the world due to its medicinal properties. ADHD and ADD are two issues that most children have been facing. A study had shown that cedar wood **can** be used to help children who have ADHD and ADD. Cedarwood is widely known for its properties to help someone calm their mind down. When applied **to** the stem of the brain, the cedarwood oil helps in releasing stress quickly.

Botanical Name – Juniperus virginiana

Color – Yellow

Perfumery Note – Base

Chamomile oil: If you are someone with a very short temper, you should use chamomile oil. This oil helps in clearing your mind and works at clearing your emotions in seconds! You will find that your emotions have stabilized when you have used chamomile oil. It clears your mind of the stress obtained through rapidly changing emotions. You will find that you can handle situations smoothly without worrying about your emotions.

Scientific Name – Matricaria chamomilla

Color – Blue

Perfumery Note - Middle

Jasmine oil: Jasmine oil is your best friend. This oil works towards keeping you confident at all times. You will find that you are more optimistic when you use this oil. If you are depressed, you will find that jasmine oil will eradicate it. You will be able to relieve your mind of any stress and will find that you can sleep better than usual.

Scientific Name – Jasminum Grandiflorum

Color – Deep brown with a tinge of gold

Perfumery Note – Base

Lavender oil: Lavender oil is the one oil that has the property of an Adaptogen. There was a study conducted in the year 1998 which had proved that people who have been using lavender oil are much more relaxed than those who do not use it. The study had also concluded that the people could solve mathematical equations even when they were drowsy. This showed that they were alert.

Scientific Name – Lavandula angustifolia

Color – Yellow

Perfumery Note – Middle

Chapter 13: Essential Oil Recipes for Stress Relief

Headache Mixture

Ingredients

- 2 Tbsp. Sweet Almond oil
- 2 Tsp. Basil oil
- 3 Tsp. Lavender oil
- 3 Tsp. Rosemary oil

Method:

- Take a dark vial and clean it completely. Allow it to dry if you have used water to clean the vial.

- Pour the oils into the vial in the order mentioned above.

- Once the oils have been poured, shake the vial well to ensure that the oils blend well. Leave this mixture overnight to let the blending happen.

- You can inhale this mixture when you have a terrible headache. This mixture will help in calming your nerves down and will also help you get rid of sinus headaches. You can also apply this oil on your forehead for faster effects.

Insomnia Relieving Blend

Ingredients:

- 2 tsp. Chamomile oil
- ½ tsp. Lavender oil
- ½ tsp. Neroli oil

Method:

- Take a small bowl and add the oils mentioned above in the same order. Mix the oils well using a spoon.

- Add some hot water in another bowl.

- Once the oils have blended well, add the oils to the hot water.

- You can inhale these vapors before you go to bed. You can also store a vial full of the oils to use every night. You will find that you can cure insomnia.

Aromatherapy bath oil blend

Ingredients:

- 8 ounces jojoba oil
- 2 Tsp. Lavender essential oil or you can use any of the oil blends mentioned above

Method:

- Take a glass bowl and clean it with a damp cloth. Once the bowl is dry, add the jojoba oil and the lavender oil to the bowl. Mix the oils well and transfer it into a vial.

- Cover the vial with an air tight stopper and leave it for a day to ensure that the oils will mix.

- Store the vial in a cool and a dark place.

- Right before you use the blend, you will need to shake the vial. Take about 8 ml of the oil and add it to the bath tub. Stir the oil well with the water with your hand to ensure that the oil and the water have mixed well.

Sleep Time Lotion

Ingredients:

- 3 ounces coconut oil
- 6 ounces liquid jojoba oil, infused
- 1-ounce bees wax, grated
- 5 Tsp. Chamomile flowers
- 5 Tsp. Lavender buds
- 8 ounces distilled water, heated
- ½ Tsp. Chamomile essential oil
- ½ Tsp. Lavender essential oil

Method:

- Take a clean glass jar and add the chamomile flowers and the lavender buds to it.

- Pour the jojoba oil to the bowl and cover the bowl and leave it aside for a few hours.

- You will need to strain the mixture and save the final product in a clean glass vial.

- You can apply this oil on your eyes or simply smell it right before you go to bed.

Grapefruit oil blend

Ingredients:

- 4 Tsp. Grapefruit oil
- 1 Tsp. Ylang Ylang oil
- 1 Tsp. Jasmine oil

Method:

- You will need to take a glass bottle and clean it with a damp cloth. When it is dry, you will need to add essential oils to the bottle.

- You will need to cover the bottle with an air tight stopper and shake the bottle well to mix the oils well.

- Keep the bottle in a cool and a dark place. You have to shake the bottle well right before you use it.

- You will need to heat the oil well and massage the oil in a circular motion to ensure that you lose the stress!

Sage oil blend

Ingredients:

- 1 tsp. lavender oil
- 1 tsp. lemon oil
- 4 tsp. sage oil

Method:

- Take a glass bottle and clean it with a damp cloth. Once it is dry, add the sage oil to it. Then add the lemon and the lavender oil to the bottle and cover it with an air tight stopper.

- Now leave the bottle in a dark place to ensure that the oils have mixed well.

- Leave the oils to blend for a day. Right before you use it, you will have to shake the bottle well.

- You will need to warm the oil a little before you use it. You will then have to massage it into your scalp.

Aromatherapy anti stress massage oil

Ingredients:

- 1 Tsp. Lavender oil
- 1 Tsp. Lemon oil
- 3 Tsp. Sage oil
- 20 ounces sweet almond oil or jojoba oil

Method:

- You will need to take a glass bottle and clean it with a damp cloth. Once the bottle is dry, you will need to add the oils to the bottle.

- You will need to cover the bottle with an air tight stopper and shake the bottle well.

- You will need to store the bottle in a dark, cool and dry place.

- Tighten the cap of the bottle and shake well.

- Right before you use the oil, you will need to shake the bottle well. You will need to use only one teaspoon of the oil to massage. Never use more than that. You could use less than that if you need.

Lavender oil blend

Ingredients:

- 1 ½ Tsp. lavender oil
- 1 Tsp. Chamomile oil
- ½ Tsp. Vetiver oil

Method:

- Take a clean glass bottle which is dark.

- Add the chamomile oil to the bottle along with the vetiver and the lavender oil.

- You will need to close the bottle with an air tight stopper and shake the oils well together to ensure that the oils mix well.

- You will need to store the bottle in a cool, dark and dry place.

- You will need to shake the bottle well before you use the blend.

- You will need to massage the oil onto your body in circular motions to obtain the best results.

Relaxing Inhalation Blend

Ingredients:

- 8 cups of boiling water
- 1 Tsp. Peppermint oil
- 1 Tsp. Eucalyptus oil
- ½ Tsp. Rosemary oil

Method:

- You will need to take a clean glass bottle. Now add the peppermint oil to the bottle.

- Now add the rosemary oil and the eucalyptus oil to the bottle and shake the bottle well to mix the oils well together.

- Take a skillet and add pour the water into the skillet. Add a few drops of the mixture of the oil to the skillet.

- You will need to cover your head with a cloth and inhale the vapor that is released. You will be able to relax and also be able to rid yourself of stress.

Relaxing Massage Oil

Ingredients:
- 56 drops of Sandalwood oil
- 40 drops of Neroli oil
- 240 drops of Rose oil

Method:

- Take a glass bottle and clean it with a damp cloth. Once it is dry, add the sandalwood oil to it. Then add the Neroli and the rose oil to the bottle and cover it with an air tight stopper.

- Now leave the bottle in a dark place to ensure that the oils have mixed well.

- Leave the oils to blend for a day. Right before you use it, you will have to shake the bottle well.

- You will need to warm the oil a little before you use it. You will then have to massage it into your scalp.

Chapter 14: A Brief Overview of Other Essential Oils

In this chapter, we are going to quickly look at a description of other common essential oils that are referenced in this book and that you might find yourself commonly using.

Anise Essential Oil: This oil possesses the distinctive aroma of black licorice. This essential oil is clear and thin. Anise essential oil is commonly used to treat bronchitis, colds, coughs, flatulence, flu, muscle aches and rheumatism.

Botanical Name – Pimpinella Anisum

Color – Clear

Perfumery Note – Top

Basil Essential Oil: This oil is an antibacterial and antiviral and also acts as an expectorant. This essential oil has a sweet, herbaceous smell. Basil essential oil is commonly used for exhaustion, gout, insect bites, sinusitis and headaches.

Botanical Name – Ocimum Basilicum

Color – Clear

Perfumery Note – Top

Cajeput Essential Oil: This essential oil is a must-have when it comes to cold and flu season. Cajeput essential oil is known for causing skin irritation and is more commonly used in a diffuser instead of for skin application. This essential oil is most commonly used to treat asthma, coughs, and sinusitis.

Botanical Name – Melaleuca Leucadendron or Melaleuca Cajupti

Color – Clear with a yellow tinge

Perfumery Note – Middle

<u>Camphor Essential Oil</u>: Camphor is an essential oil that is able to be used for many purposes. Camphor is effective to facilitate digestion and blood circulation, relieve gas troubles, cure inflammation, provide relief from spasms and cramps, and relieve congestion in both the nasal tracts and lungs, works as an insecticide, germicide and disinfectant. Camphor essential oil is also known to reduce the severity of nervous disorders, aid in the treatment of food poisoning and bug bites, boosts libido and helps to cure erectile problems.

Botanical Name – Cinnamomum Camphora and Laurus Camphora

Color – White

Perfumery Note – Middle

195

Cardamom Essential Oil: This essential oil is uplifting and energizing. It is typically used by those who are challenged with stress, fatigue, depression and despair. Known as an aphrodisiac, cardamom essential oil is also used to treat loss of appetite, colic, and halitosis

Botanical Name – Elettaria Cardamomum

Color – Clear

Perfumery Note – Middle

Cinnamon Essential Oil: This essential oil is much richer in aroma than the cinnamon we would purchase at the store. Cinnamon essential oil is used to treat constipation, exhaustion, flatulence, lice, low blood pressure, scabies and stress.

Botanical Name – Cinnamomum Zeylanicum

Color – Golden yellow to brown

Perfumery Note – Middle

<u>Citronella Essential Oil</u>: This oil is well known to be a repellent against mosquitoes and other insects. Citronella essential oil is also known to help against excessive perspiration, fatigue, headache, and oily skin.

Botanical Name – Cymbopogon Nardus / Cymbopogon Winterianus

Color – Clear

Perfumery Note – Top

<u>Grapefruit Essential Oil</u>: This essential oil is an energizing oil that isn't overwhelming in scent. Some of the uses for grapefruit essential oil include minimizing cellulitis, brightening dull skin, and eliminating both toxins build up and water retention. Grapefruit is considered to be a phototoxic essential oil and must be used with caution when applying to the skin.

Botanical Name – Citrus Paradisi

Color – Pale yellow to medium yellow

Perfumery Note - Top

Jasmine Essential Oil: Jasmine blossoms cannot be effectively steam distilled, so they are extracted by a solvent to create a highly concentrated absolute, which means a tiny bit of this essential oil goes a long way. Jasmine essential oil is used to treat depression, dry skin, exhaustion, and labor pains. Jasmine is also a good choice for those who suffer from sensitive skin.

Botanical Name – Jasminum Grandiflorum

Color – Deep brown with a golden tinge

Perfumery Note – Middle

Juniper Essential Oil: This essential oil is a natural antiseptic. It is used to combat acne when it is used in low dilutions for skin care application. Juniper essential oil can also be used as a room mist or air freshener which helps to kill airborne germs. Some other uses for juniper essential oil include treating colds, flu, acne, cellulitis, gout, hemorrhoids, and rheumatism.

Botanical Name – Juniperus Communis

Color – Clear

Perfumery Note – Middle

Lime Essential Oil: This essential oil falls under the citrus category of essential oils. The interesting thing about lime essential oil is that it isn't always phototoxic. When you choose distilled lime essential oil instead of cold pressed lime essential oil it is not phototoxic. Lime essential oil is commonly used as a room freshener or to treat acne, dull skin and varicose veins.

Botanical Name – Citrus Aurantifolia

Color – Light green with a hint of orange or yellow.

Perfumery Note – Top

Nutmeg Essential Oil: This essential oil has a rich, woody scent similar to the scent of the cooking spice, but a little richer and more fragrant. Nutmeg essential oil is commonly used to treat arthritis, constipation, fatigue, muscle aches, nausea, poor circulation and slow digestion.

Botanical Name – Myristica Fragrans

Color – Clear

Perfumery Note – Middle

Oak Moss Essential Oil: This essential oil is extracted through solvent extraction which makes it an absolute. Oak moss essential oil is most commonly used in perfumery. It is known for its earthy aroma and its properties as a fragrance fixative.

Botanical Name – Evernia Prunastri

Color – Dark Brown

Perfumery Note – Base

Orange Essential Oil: This oil is known as being versatile and affordable. Orange essential oil is one of the most popular oils in aromatherapy. It is great for helping to improve the aroma of a stale-smelling or smoky room, and it is also commonly used in cleaning products. Orange essential oil is also commonly used to treat colds, constipation, dull skin, flatulence, slow digestion and stress.

Botanical Name – Citrus Sinesis

Color – Greenish Orange

Perfumery Note – Top

Oregano Essential Oil: This essential oil is well known for its herbaceous and sharp smell. While not as common as some of the other essential oils, oregano essential oil is beneficial when treating coughs or aiding digestion.

Botanical Name – Oreganum Vulgare

Color – Pale yellow

Perfumery Note - Medium

Peppermint Essential Oil: The aroma of peppermint is well-known to most people. While a favorite around Christmas time, peppermint essential oil is popular year-round to ease tension headaches and enhance alertness and stamina. Peppermint essential oil is considered an aphrodisiac and is commonly used to treat exhaustion, nausea, sinusitis, and vertigo.

Botanical Name – Mentha Piperita

Color – Clear with a yellow tinge

Perfumery Note – Top

Pine Essential Oil: Another favorite to be used around Christmas time, pine essential oil is a medium to a strong aroma that is commonly used in diffusers. Pine essential oil is effective at treating coughs, colds, flu, and sinusitis.

Botanical Name – Pinus Sylvestris

Color – Clear

Perfumery Note – Middle

Spearmint Essential Oil: This essential oil is similar to peppermint essential oil, but has a subtler scent. Many people choose to replace some or all of the peppermint essential oil in a recipe with spearmint to help tone down the smell.

Botanical Name – Mentha Spicata or Mentha Cardiaca

Color – Clear

Perfumery Note – Top

Thyme Essential Oil: Historically, fresh and dried thyme, as well as thyme essential oil have been used to help ward off bacteria and viruses. Some of the more common uses for thyme essential oil are arthritis, colds, cuts, flu, insect bites, lice, muscle aches, poor circulation, scabies and sore throat.

Botanical Name – Thymus Vulgaris or Thymus Zygis

Color – Pale yellow, although it can be varied depending on the specific botanic and distillation used.

Perfumery Note - Middle

Vanilla Essential Oil: Most people are familiar with the scent of vanilla. Vanilla essential oil is most commonly solvent extracted which makes it an absolute. Vanilla essential oil is commonly used in perfumery and to enhance the fragrance of aromatherapy and skin and hair care formulations.

Botanical Name – Vanilla Planifolia

Color – Deep brown

Perfumery Note – Base

Vetiver Essential Oil: This essential oil can be used for both topical and fragrant applications. Topically, it is commonly used to treat acne, oily skin, cuts, muscular aches, and sores. When used as aromatherapy it is used to treat depression, exhaustion, insomnia, and stress.

Botanical Name – Vetiveria Zizanoides

Color – Golden brown to dark brown

Perfumery Note – Base

Chapter 15: Essential Oil Recipes for General Skin Care

In this chapter, we are going to take a look at some more essential oil recipes that are great for the skin all over your body. We are going to look at some recipes for stretch marks, moisturizing, eczema and even soap.

Body Butter for Varicose Veins: This body butter is a great option to help subdue the effects of varicose veins. To make this recipe you are going to use a double boiler on medium-low and stir the Shea butter and coconut oil for a few minutes until it melts. Once it has melted, you are going to add the rest of the ingredients and place it in the fridge for an hour. After an hour, mix with a hand mixer for about ten minutes until you have soft white peaks. You can store this in a glass container for about six months. Use daily, in the morning.

The ingredients:

- Five (5) drops of cypress essential oil

- Five (5) drops of lemon essential oil

- Ten (10) drops of fennel essential oil

- Ten (10) drops of helichrysum essential oil

- One-quarter (1/4) of a cup jojoba oil

- One-quarter (1/4) of a cup coconut oil

- One-half (1/2) of a cup of Shea butter

Body Scrubs: The body scrub recipes below are great replacements for soaps. They exfoliate your skin and can easily be modified to your personal skin needs and preferences. To make these recipes, simply combine the ingredients and store in a glass container.

Body Scrub Recipe for Sensitive Skin:

- Four (4) drops of lavender essential oil

- Three (3) drops of roman chamomile essential oil

- Three (3) drops of geranium essential oil

- One and a half (1 ½) cups of sea salt

- One-quarter (1/4) of a cup of coconut oil

Body Scrub Recipe for Oily Skin

- Five (5) drops of tea tree essential oil

- Five (5) drops of rosemary essential oil

- One and a half (1 ½) cups of ground coffee

- One-quarter (1/4) of a cup of jojoba oil

Body Scrub Recipe for Dry Skin with Eczema

- Four (4) drops of lavender essential oil

- Three (3) drops of carrot seed essential oil

- Three (3) drops of neroli essential oil

- One and a half (1 ½) cups of sugar

- One-quarter (1/4) of a cup of olive oil

Stretch Mark Serum: This serum is a great option for providing nourishment and hydration, fading and preventing stretch marks, rebuilding collagen, increasing circulation and elasticity. Use this oil once or twice a day for a few months to reduce the appearance of stretch marks and scars.

In a glass container, mix:

- Five (5) drops of neroli essential oil

- Five (5) drops of lavender essential oil

- Five (5) drops of myrrh essential oil

- Five (5) drops of lemon essential oil

- Two (2) tablespoons of vitamin E oil

- Two (2) tablespoons of rosehip oil

- Two (2) tablespoons of jojoba oil

Chapter 16: Best Essential Oils for Weight Loss

Essential oils do not help in weight loss alone. We need to address a holistic approach when it comes to weight loss. It is our health that we must factor when we are looking at losing weight. We need to change our diet and our lifestyle along with the use of essential oils.

You must know that most essential oils that are used in aiding weight loss also have an impact on our emotions. The oils are used to help give us a positive image of ourselves and our body. They help us connect with our bodies and nurture us from within.

It is possible to use essential oils individually, but it is best to use a blend of equal proportions of these oils.

They help in giving us the perfect balance and help us therapeutically. Essential oils stated below work wonders when it comes to weight loss.

Grapefruit: Grapefruit oil is commonly used as an antiseptic. It is used as a disinfectant too. It helps get rid of excess water retention in your body. It increases energy and curbs your hunger pangs. It helps reduce the fat accumulated around the abdomen. Grapefruit contains a natural chemical compound called Nootaktone. It is this that helps in losing body fat. Grapefruit also contains limonene which allows the body to release fatty acids into the blood which in turn increases energy.

Grapefruit is a perfect aid for weight loss. It helps in reducing the quantity of cellulite in your body. It helps your urge to overeat and also helps in toning the muscles. It reduces the stress that one feels because of the strict weight loss regime. It also helps in boosting your self – image and helps you accept yourself for the person you are.

A couple of drops of grapefruit oil (which is consumable) when added to a glass of water and had on waking up every morning helps in losing weight.

Botanical Name – Citrus paradisi

Color – Pale Yellow or Light Ruby

Perfumery Note – Top

Lemon: The oil from a lemon helps in detoxifying the body. It increases the energy levels of the body and also gets rid of parasites that are in the intestines. It helps in reducing the number of digestive disorders that could occur. On an emotional level, it helps in reducing the intensity of your judgment towards you.

Botanical Name – Citrus Limon

Color – Pale yellow to deep yellow

Perfumery Note - Top

Peppermint: Peppermint is any man's best friend if he is on a weight loss regime. It is known to relieve you of depression and any other heavy emotions. It boosts your confidence and increases the level of optimism. It also helps in ridding your body of multiple digestive issues.

Peppermint oil is known to help in digestion and reduce bloating. It also relaxes the muscles and makes you feel less hungry. It is also known to increase energy and keep you alert. This oil is loaded with nutrients that are very beneficial for your body. Inhaling this oil itself helps curb your craving for food. If you find the smell too strong to inhale, you can add about 3 - 4 of drops of the oil to a glass of water and drink it. It reduces your appetite. You can also add a few drops of it to your water bath.

Botanical Name – Mentha x Piperita

Color – Clear to Pale Yellow

Perfumery Note – Top

Ginger: Ginger oil is a liquid psychiatrist. It helps in increasing your willingness to change your attitude. It helps in empowering you and increases your inner strength. It is known to help in digestion and also aid in curing digestive issues. It helps in increasing the energy in the body and also helps in stimulating the entire digestive system to burn the extra fat.

Botanical Name – Zingiber Officinale

Color – Light Yellow

Perfumery Note – Middle to base

Bergamot oil: Bergamot oil is obtained from Italian citrus fruits. Bergamot oil is known to increase energy and cure depression. It is a stress buster. It is a mood booster. People who are obese are depressed, so bergamot oil helps cure depression and stress. It is heart healthy too.

A couple of drops of this oil when poured on a handkerchief and inhaled help you feel relaxed and revitalized. A few drops mixed with coconut oil and massaged on the feet and neck will help you.

Botanical Name – Citrus bergamia

Color – Green to Yellow

Perfumery Note – Top to Middle

Cinnamon oil: This oil is obtained from the inner bark of the Cinnamomum tree. It may be obtained from the leaves too. It can regulate blood sugar levels in the body. When your body becomes insulin resistant, you end up gaining weight, and your blood sugar levels may rise. It helps to boost the immune system. Blood circulation is improved. It also cures people who have irritable bowel syndrome. Cinnamon oil is known to improve insulin sensitivity.

Inhaling this oil a few minutes before your meals helps control your food intake. You can also have 4-5 drops of it in a glass of water either early morning or just before you sleep at night.

Botanical Name – Cinnamomum Verum

Color – Yellow to red brown

Perfumery Note – Top

Fennel oil: This oil is obtained from fennel seeds which are steam distilled. It curbs your hunger and improves your digestion. It helps in controlling weight gain. It also gives you peaceful sleep.

Botanical Name – Foeniculum vulgare

Color – Green

Perfumery Note – Middle to Top

Lemongrass oil: Oil is taken out from the stalks. Apart from helping you to lose weight, lemongrass oil also helps in acne and aches.

Botanical Name – Cymbopogon Citratus or Cymbopogon Flecuosus

Color – Pale yellow to vivid yellow

Perfumery Note – Top

Rosemary oil: This oil is obtained from the rosemary plant and is known to help you lose fat.

Botanical Name – Rosmarinus officinalis

Color – Clear

Perfumery Note – Middle

Spearmint oil: Spearmint oil is known to help in digestion and reduce bloating. It also relaxes the muscle and makes you feel less hungry. It is also known to increase energy and keep you alert. It also helps to cure fever.

Other oils that may help in weight loss are tangerine oil, clove oil, sandalwood oil, orange oil, patchouli oil, celery seed oil, Ylang Ylang oil, etc.

Botanical Name – Mentha spicata

Color – Pink

Perfumery Note – Top

Chapter 17: Essential Oil Recipes for Weight Loss

Appetite Suppressant

Ingredients:

- 1 Tsp. Ginger root oil
- 2 Tsp. Lemon oil
- Four Tsp. Mandarin oil
- 1 Tsp. Peppermint oil

Method:

- Take a clean glass vial and add the oils in the order mentioned above.

- Cover the vial with an air tight stopper and shake the vial gently.

- You will need to add a few drops of this blend to your diffuser before you use it.

Metabolism Boosting Bath Soak

Ingredients:

- 1 Tsp. Cypress oil
- 1 Tsp. Grapefruit oil
- 1 Tsp. rosemary oil
- ½ cup jojoba oil

Method:

- Take a clean glass bottle or a jar and add essential oils to the jar.

- Cover the jar with an air tight stopper and shake the jar well to ensure that the oils blend.

- You will need to store the jar in a cool and a dark place till you use the mixture.

- You will need to add 2 tbsp. of the mixture to your bath with warm water. You will need to mix the water well with your hands.

- You could stay in the tub for an hour.

Anti-Cellulite Balm

Ingredients:

- ½ Tsp. Cypress oil
- ½ Tsp. Ginger oil
- 3 Tsp. Grapefruit oil
- ½ Tsp. Peppermint oil
- 1 Tsp. rosemary oil
- 4 Tbsp. almond oil at every use

Method:

- You will need to take a large glass mixing bowl and clean it with a damp cloth. You will need to let the bowl dry.

- Once it is dry add all essential oils except for the almond oil.

- Transfer the blend into a clean dark glass vial and cover it with an air tight stopper.

- Store this vial in a cool place.

- Right before you use it, you will need to pour ½ tbsp. Of the almond oil into a bowl along with 20 drops of the essential oil. Mix it well and massage the oil lightly onto your skin.

Massage oil for weight loss

Ingredients:
- 1 Tsp. cypress oil
- 1 Tsp. grapefruit oil
- 1 Tsp. lemon oil
- 2 cups almond oil

Method:

- Take a glass bottle and clean it with a damp cloth and leave it to dry.

- Add the almond oil to the glass bottle a followed by the remaining essential oils. Shake the bottle well to ensure that the oils have blended well with each other.

- You will need to store the bottle in a cold and a dark place.

- Right before you use the oil, you will need to massage it in the area where you want the fat to reduce. You will have to massage well to have your body absorb the oil.

Citrus Weight Loss Inhaler

Ingredients:

- 4 Tsp. Grapefruit oil
- ¼ Tsp. Lemon oil
- ¼ Tsp. Ylang Ylang oil
- 4 Tsp. coarse sea salt

Method:

- Take a medium sized glass bowl and add the salt to the bowl.

- Now pour the grapefruit oil and mix the oil and the salt.

- Next, add the remaining oils to the bowl and mix them all.

- Transfer the blend to a glass vial and leave it in a cold and a dark place. Make sure that the place is dry.

- You will only have to sniff this oil between deep breaths. You will need to breathe the scent in twice to ensure that there is a good effect of the oil on your body.

Belly Busting massage oil

Ingredients:

- 1 Tsp. cypress oil
- 1 Tsp. grapefruit oil
- 1 Tsp. Juniper berry oil
- ½ Tsp. Sage oil
- 1 Tsp. sweet orange oil
- 10 ounces almond oil

Method:

- Take a clean glass bowl and add the almond oil to the bowl.

- Add the remaining essential oils to the bowl and mix them well.

- Transfer the oil blend into a glass vial and cover it well with an air tight stopper and store it in a dark place.

- Right before you use the oil, you will need to shake the vial well. Take 2 – 3 tbsp. Of the blend and warm it before you apply it on the area where you want to lose the fat. You will need to massage the oil for a minimum of half an hour. You should not remove the oil. Let your body absorb it.

Detox drink

Ingredients:

- 4 cups distilled water

- ¼ Tsp. Lemon oil
- ¼ Tsp. Grapefruit oil
- ½ cup fresh grapefruit juice
- A few drops stevia to taste

Method:

- Take a glass vial or a jar and add the ingredients to the vial.

- Cover the vial with an air tight container.

- Leave the vial in the refrigerator and consume only one teaspoon a day.

Curb Craving Balm

Ingredients:

- 1 Tsp. bergamot oil
- 2 Tsp. Fennel oil
- ½ Tsp. Patchouli oil
- 8 Tbsp. olive oil

Method:

- Take a glass bowl and add the ingredients in the order mentioned above.

- Mix the oils well together and transfer the ingredients to a glass vial and shake it well.

- You will need to massage the oil on your abdomen in a circular motion. Do not wash off the oil but let your body absorb it.

Chapter 18: Essential Oils for Other Health Benefits

The beauty care treatments that we have covered in the previous chapters are just the tip of the ice burg when it comes to all of the uses that essential oils have. In this chapter, we are going to look at some of the other health benefits you can get from using essential oils.

Migraine Headache Relief – To help ease the pain of headaches, you can combine a few drops of lavender essential and peppermint essential oil and apply it to your temples to help with headaches and migraines.

<u>Reduce Cough Or Sinusitis</u> – Eucalyptus oil is known for its powerful ability to fight coughs and open airways. Adding a few drops of steaming water or a diffuser and inhaling will help to clear your nasal passage.

<u>Repair Broken Bones</u> – It might seem a little far-fetched to think that an essential oil can help with the repair of broken bones. However, helichrysum, fir and cypress essential oils all contain properties that support the healing of broken bones.

<u>Heal Burns</u> – It is well known that Aloe Vera is effective in treating burns. However, if you mix a few drops of lavender into your Aloe Vera, it will treat burns more effectively.

Soothe Bug Bites – Lavender essential oil is also an effective option for treating any bug bites and stings. It will take the itch and the stinging out.

Improve Digestion – A combination of ginger essential oil, peppermint essential oil, and fennel essential oils aids in support of digestion and helps to heal a leaky gut.

Asthma Rub – A combination of eucalyptus and peppermint essential oils combined with coconut oils makes a homemade vapor rub that helps to open up the lungs.

Treat Bruises – Adding essential oils to a hot compress can help to treat bruises and other wounds. Simply add five drops of lavender and five drops of frankincense to four ounces of hot water and soak a cotton cloth in the mixture. Apply to the affected area.

Improve Concentration – Inhaling bergamot, grapefruit, or peppermint essential oils can help to increase your concentration throughout the day.

Sore Feet Soak – Adding ten drops of peppermint essential oil and a tablespoon of Epsom salts to a warm water foot bath will help to ease your foot pain and relax you.

Reduce Teeth Grinding – If you find that you wake up with a sore jaw from grinding your teeth while you are asleep massage one to three drops of lavender essential oil to the bottom of your feet and behind your ears before you go to bed to help reduce the amount you are grinding your teeth.

Relieve PMS – Mix two drops each of sage, basil, and rosemary. Apply this mixture to a warm, moist hand towel and apply the warm towel to your abdomen.

Improve Circulation – Add eight to ten drops of grapefruit essential oil to warm bath water. Combine in the water and enjoy a good soak in the bath.

Relieve Hangover Symptoms – To help ease your hangover symptoms, add six drops each of juniper berry, cedar wood, rosemary, grapefruit, lavender, and lemon essential oils in to a warm bath.

Curb Food Cravings – Inhaling peppermint and cinnamon essential oils can help to reduce your appetite and balance your blood sugars.

Energize Your Workout – To help reduce the fatigue you feel while you are working out, inhale peppermint essential oil before beginning.

Reduce Fever – If you find yourself with a fever, add one to three drops each of eucalyptus, peppermint, and lavender to a cool cloth and sponge the body.

Relieve Motion Sickness – To help reduce the effects of motion sickness, use a mixture of peppermint, lavender and ginger essential oils.

Arthritis Relief – You can relieve the pain felt from arthritis if you mix two drops each of wintergreen, cypress, and lemongrass essential oils into an unscented lotion. Massage the lotion into affected areas.

Treat Ringworm – Combine three drops of tea tree essential oil with coconut oil and massage over the area affected by ringworm twice a day.

Treat Head Lice – To treat head lice, mix three drops each of thyme, lavender, and eucalyptus essential oils with unscented oil and apply to the scalp. Cover head with a shower cap and leave on your head for thirty minutes. Shampoo the mixture off of your scalp.

Heal Blistered Skin – If you are suffering from blistered skin, mix two drops of tea tree essential oil with two drops of an unscented oil and apply to the blistered area up to five times per day.

Soothe A Sunburn – If you find yourself with a sunburn, combine lavender or chamomile essential oil with one tablespoon of coconut oil. Apply this mixture to the skin with a cotton ball to reduce swelling and pain.

Treat Poison Ivy – If you have suffered a run-in with poison oak or poison ivy, mix three drops of peppermint essential oil with unscented oil and apply to the affected area.

Lose Weight – To help support your metabolism, mix grapefruit, ginger and cinnamon essential oils and take as a supplement three times a day.

Boost Immune System – If you are going to be travelling by plane and want to boost your immune system, mix one drop of oregano essential oil with four drops of a carrier oil and rub on the bottom of your feet before flying.

Improve Allergies – You don't need to suffer from itchy eyes and throat when you find yourself hit with allergies. Rub Frankincense and lavender essential oils on your palms and inhale deeply.

There are many other uses for essential oils in your life to replace other products you are using right now that could be affecting your health. In the next chapter, we are going to look at why most products you are using might not be the best products for you and how you can replace those products with homemade products using essential oils.

Chapter 19: Essential Oils around the House

Many of the commercial products you are using in your home are made with synthetically made chemicals. In fact, many of these products are labelled to say that they are hazardous to humans and domestic animals! While we want to get products that are going to clean our home, we shouldn't be doing this at the cost of our health or the environment. The good news is that we can replace many of the products in our home with natural options using essential oils. One major advantage of using essential oils is that you can get the benefits of a clean home along with a boost to your mind and body wellness.

In this chapter, we are going to look at some of the products in our homes that we can replace with essential oil recipes.

245

Cleaning Your Floors

When it comes to cleaning your floors, you want something that is going to lift dirt, take out stains and remove odors.

To Wash Floors – Fills a large container with one gallon of hot water. Add two to four tablespoons of Castile soap and ten drops of lemon essential oil. Stir the mixture and wash your floors as you normally would.

To Clean Carpets – Mix twenty drops of tea tree essential oil with Borax. Sprinkle over your carpets and let sit for ten to fifteen minutes. Vacuum carpets like you usually would.

Cleaning Your Bathroom

Everyone wants a clean bathroom. When you think about what happens in the bathroom, it is important that you have cleaning supplies that are going to leave your bathroom disinfected and smelling good.

Toilet Cleaning – Add two cups of water and two teaspoons of tea tree essential oil to a spray bottle. Give it a good shake and spray into the toilet's rim. Let the mixture sit for about thirty minutes before scrubbing.

Eliminate Shower Curtain Scum – Mix four drops of eucalyptus essential oil with four drops of tea tree essential oil. Add to a spray bottle with warm water. Spray onto your shower curtain for natural mold killing action.

Bathtub Scrub – Mix one-half of a cup of baking soda with one-half of a cup of vinegar. Add five drops of bergamot or lime essential oil. Use the mixture as a scrub for your sink or bathtub.

Bathroom Freshener – Soak a cotton ball soaked in lime or lemon essential oil behind the toilet to use as a bathroom freshener.

Cleaning Your Kitchen

Counter Cleaner – Add three drops each of lemon essential oil and tea tree essential oil to a few ounces of warm water. Mix into a spray bottle and spray countertops and cutting boards to naturally disinfect them.

Cleaning Burnt Pans – Add a few drops of lemon essential oil to and some boiling water to help remove burnt on foods from your pots and pans.

Freshen Your Trash Can – Place two drops each of lemon essential oil and tea tree essential oil onto a cotton ball. Place the cotton ball at the bottom of the trashcan to help decrease the odor and detoxify the air.

Clear The Air Of Strong Cooking Odors – Add a few drops of clove, cinnamon, or citrus essential oils to a pan of simmering water to get rid of odors in the air left from cooking.

Purify Fridge – To leave your fridge smelling great after you wash it out, add a few drops of lime, grapefruit or bergamot essential oils to the water you use to rinse your fridge.

Cleaner Dishes – Instead of using commercial dishwashing detergent, make your own dishwasher pods. In a bowl, mix two teaspoons each of tangerine and lemon essential oils. Add one-half of a cup of kosher salt and one-half of a cup of white vinegar. Next, add two cups of Borax and two cups of washing soda. Using an ice cube tray, portion out the mixture and allow the pods to dry for twenty-four to forty-eight hours. Once the pods are dry, remove them from the tray and store in an air tight container. Use one pod per cycle.

Add a few drops of lemon essential oil to the dishwasher before washing dishes for a spot free rinse.

Around The Home

Sports gear – There is nothing worse than the smell of sports gear coated in sweat. Add two drops of tea tree essential oil to one quart of warm water, next add four tablespoons of baking soda and mix well. Use this mixture to clean jerseys, cleats and other sports gear.

Washing Machine – Using a box grater, grate one bar of Castile soap. In a bowl, mix the soap with two cups of Borax, two cups of washing soda, three teaspoons each of lavender and tea tree essential oils and one teaspoon of lemon essential oil. Mix until a damp powder is formed. Store in an airtight container and use one-quarter of a cup for each regular load of laundry.

Add ten to twenty drops of your favorite essential oil to your washing machine each time you do a load of laundry.

Washing Produce – To clean fruits and vegetables naturally, add two drops of lemon essential oil to a large bowl of water and then wash.

Eliminate Smoke – To remove the smell of cigarette smoke from your home or car, put four drops each of rosemary, tea tree and eucalyptus essential oils to a spray bottle of water and spray as needed.

Reduce Paint Fumes – Add a couple of drops of peppermint and eucalyptus essential oils to a gallon of paint to help dispel the fumes.

Bad Smelling Shoes – To remove the smell from shoes, add a few drops of tea tree essential oil and lemon essential oil to freshen them up.

Clean Windows – Mix two ounces of water and ten drops of lavender essential oil in a spray bottle. Spritz on your windows and wipe them clean to get rid of grime and ward off flies.

Furniture Polish – Combine four ounces of jojoba oil with twelve drops of lemon essential oil, eight drops of sandalwood essential oil, and four drops of lemongrass essential oil in a spray bottle. Shake up the mixture and apply onto a cloth and use it to wipe wood surfaces.

Chapter 20: Essential Oils and Aromatherapy

Now that we have looked at many of the physical applications of essential oils and how they can benefit you, we are going to look at the inhalation of essential oils and the benefits that inhaling the oils can bring. Before we get into that information, let's have a look at what aromatherapy is and how it can benefit you.

Aromatherapy is an alternative medicine that uses essential oils to improve a person's health or mood. While many people consider this type of treatment to be unscientific and wishful thinking, there have been some scientific studies showing that aromatherapy is effective at making you feel good, although there was no evidence that it makes you well.

Essential oils that are used in aromatherapy have a different composition than other herbal products you can purchase. This is because the distillation that happens in aromatherapy recovers the lighter phytol molecules.

History of Aromatherapy

Aromatherapy is not a practice that has just been invented. It is an age old practice that has come into the limelight only in the recent decade. The tradition of using aromatherapy started during the birth of Jesus Christ. This would imply that the process of aromatherapy was invented 4000 years ago. There are many civilizations over the years that have used the oils of different plants like cinnamon, ginger, sandalwood, rose and lavender. They had extracted these oils for the medicinal properties that they contain.

Aromatherapy has deep roots in India as well! It has been mentioned in the literature of Early Indian Medicine. It was 4000 years ago when the Indians had listed the medicinal properties of the oils of 700 plants! These oils were then called essential oils. Ayurveda, which is the traditional Indian medicine, uses aromatic massages as a therapy to treat patients. These massages used the oils that were extracted from the different plants. It is only recently that the aromatic massages have become popular across the world, especially in the West.

The Chinese took the use of essential oils a step further. They used the oils to cure a variety of illnesses! A Chinese practitioner and pharmacist, Shen Nung had written a book about the different herbs that could be used to cure diseases. This is the oldest Chinese book to have the information of 400 plants and their medicinal properties. It was during this time that the Egyptians had also begun to use essential oils. They had begun to master the art of aromatherapy. They used to extract the oils from the different herbs and plants around them. They used these oils to help them cure illnesses. They also used to burn wood that had great fragrances and shows their respect to the Gods they worshipped.

The Egyptians, however, took aromatherapy a step further! They used to use the oils they extracted from Chamomile and Galbanum to cleanse the bodies of the Pharaohs. This was done before they were embalmed. When they have created the case for the Pharaoh, they also placed Cinnamon, Myrrh and Cassia oils in the case. The Pharaohs were wrapped in a separate cloth. This cloth was saturated in the oils of cinnamon, cedarwood, juniper, and myrrh. The body of the Pharaoh was also rubbed in essential oils. These oils were used to preserve the body for life after death. There were some wealthy Egyptians who had used essential oils in their baths, for skin care and also as lotions. The Romans and the Greeks were not far behind. They, like the Egyptians, mastered the art of aromatherapy. They had begun to use essential oils in their medicines and also as cosmetics.

It is over the last few years that Aromatherapy has gained importance. You may still be wondering what it is all about. But, the fact is that spas and salons are offering the best massages! They have tried to cater to the needs of the people. This could be either physical or psychological. The spas have multiple aromatic therapies. These therapies are what help in reducing the stress that they may have been feeling all day! They could come there to be treated like the kings and queens of the world! The aromatic therapies that are used in these spas are the treatments that have been developed in ancient Rome, Greece, and Egypt. There are quite a few hotels across the world that allows you to be pampered in a spa!

How Does Aromatherapy Work?

It is commonly believed that the inhalation of essential oils stimulates the olfactory system, which is the part of the brain that is connected to smell. When this happens, a signal is sent to the limbic system of the brain that is responsible for controlling emotions and retrieves learned memories which lead to memories to be released which will make a person feel relaxed, happy, calm, or even stimulated.

When we target our sense of smell with essential oils, we are being affected emotionally. When we apply essential oils topically, we are activating thermal receptors and destroying microbes and fungi.

When you are using your essential oils topically, you are still taking advantage of the aromatherapy benefits that come with essential oils.

Benefits of Inhaling Essential Oils

When essential oils are inhaled into the lungs, it brings both physical and psychological benefits. Here is a brief list of the benefits that can be found by inhaling essential oils along with essential oils that can be used for each purpose.

1. Stress Relief:

- Lavender essential oil

- Frankincense essential oil

- Rose essential oil

- Roman Chamomile essential oil

- Vanilla essential oil

2. Sinus Congestion Relief:

- Tea Tree essential oil
- Eucalyptus essential oil
- Lavender essential oil
- Peppermint essential oil
- Oregano essential oil

3. Sore Throat Relief:

- Eucalyptus essential oil
- Rosemary essential oil
- Camphor essential oil
- Thyme essential oil
- Sage essential oil

4. <u>Cough Relief</u>:

- Tea tree essential oil

- Myrrh essential oil

- Peppermint essential oil

- Lavender essential oil

- Lemon essential oil

5. <u>Bronchitis Relief</u>:

- Lavender essential oil

- Frankincense essential oil

- Eucalyptus essential oil

- Peppermint essential oil

6. <u>Anxiety Relief</u>:

- Bergamot essential oil

- Frankincense essential oil

- Basil essential oil

- Sage essential oil

- Lavender essential oil

- Marjoram essential oil

- Ylang-ylang essential oil

7. <u>Depression Relief</u>:

- Lavender essential oil

- Rose essential oil

- Geranium essential oil

- Bergamot essential oil

- Sandalwood essential oil

- Marjoram essential oil

- Jasmine essential oil

8. Insomnia Relief:

- Lavender essential oil

- Marjoram essential oil

- Neroli essential oil

- Roman Chamomile essential oil

- Ylang-ylang essential oil

How to Inhale Essential Oils

When you decide to begin inhaling essential oils, it is important to make sure that you are doing it correctly. There are a few different ways that you can inhale your favorite oils, all of which will get the compounds of your oil into your throat, lungs and blood stream.

1. <u>A Few Drops By Your Pillow</u>: Inhalation works best when it is given time to work. This is why placing essential oils on your pillow or a cotton ball near your pillow is an effective option. Simply place three to five drops of the essential oil of your choice onto the corner of your pillow or a cotton ball.

2. <u>On a Tissue/Pocket Square/Handkerchief</u>: This option is great if you are treating a cold. Simply place one to three drops of the essential oil on your favorite tissue and you will be able to carry it around with you and inhale liberally.

3. Using an Aromatherapy Inhaler: This is a small option, similar to a tobacco vaporizer. To use, simply add your preferred essential oil to the insert that is included, slide it into the plastic inhaler tube and seal it with the cap.

4. Steam Inhalation: If you are relaxing at home, this is a great relaxing option. Simply pour some hot water into a bowl and add two to three drops of your chosen essential oil and stir thoroughly. Cover your head with a towel and lean your face about ten inches over the steaming bowl for one to two minutes, with your eyes closed. Take deep breaths through your nose and repeat two to four times, as necessary.

5. Using an Essential Oil Diffuser: This method is the least efficient if you are trying to clear a congestion or similar ailment. However, if you are looking for stress, depression, anxiety or insomnia relief, investing in an essential oil diffuser is a very good idea.

When you are using any of the above methods, you can blend essential oils as you wish to, to create a personalized smell that is exactly what you want and need for your personal situation.

Risks to Aromatherapy

As with anything, there are some risks to using aromatherapy. There are some instances when you should be extra cautious as you explore aromatherapy:

- If you have any allergies;

- If you suffer from hay fever;

- If you suffer from asthma; or

- If you have any skin conditions such as eczema or psoriasis.

You must be extremely cautious with aromatherapy and essential oils if:

- You suffer from epilepsy;

- You suffer from hypertension;

- You have deep vein thrombosis;

- You are breastfeeding; or

- You are pregnant.

Occasionally you might experience some side effects from using aromatherapy. The side effects can include nausea, headaches and some allergic reactions. However, the reactions tend to be very mild and do not   last   long.

Chapter 21: Aromatherapy Blends

In the last chapter, we covered the different essential oils that can be used when you choose to inhale essential oils. However, you aren't limited to using only one essential oil in these methods. You can also create blends that you can place on your pillow, in a diffuser, or in any of the other methods. For each of the blends, combine in a dark colored glass bottle. For these blends, you do not need carrier oil unless you are applying them to the skin.

Insomnia Aromatherapy Blend:

- Ten (10) drops of roman chamomile essential oil

- Five (5) drops of sage essential oil

- Five (5) drops of bergamot essential oil

Anxiety Aromatherapy Blend:

- Ten (10) drops of bergamot essential oil

- Ten (10) drops of sage essential oil

- Five (5) drops of frankincense essential oil

Stress Relieving Aromatherapy Blend:

- Ten (10) drops of roman chamomile essential oil

- Five (5) drops of lavender essential oil

Depression Aromatherapy Blend:

- Ten (10) drops of grapefruit essential oil

- Five (5) drops of ylang-ylang essential oil

- Five (5) drops of lavender essential oil

Congestion Aromatherapy Blend:

- Thirty (30) drops of eucalyptus essential oil

- Twenty-Six (26) drops of myrrh essential oil

- Four (4) drops of peppermint essential oil

Chapter 22: A Few Notes on Creating Your Own Essential Oil Recipes

Now that you have some knowledge of which essential oils are best for what, you are by no means limited to the recipes we have shown you. In this chapter, we are going to show you how you can start creating your blends and recipes.

Blending your essential oils can save you a lot of money because you aren't going to have to spend money on purchasing a blend that someone else has prepared. Creating your own blends is a combination of creativity and science, and there are a few things you should know about it.

When you create a blend to achieve a purpose, you probably don't want a blend that has an unappealing scent. Next, we are going to cover some tips on how to create blends that smell good.

Keep in mind; traditional perfumers that work for the famous fragrance houses study for years in order to master the art and science of perfumery blending. It is going to take some trial and error before you are able to accurately predict what is going to accomplish a particular smell.

Blending Basics

Essential oils can be categorized into broad groups based on their aroma. To get you started here is a list of some of the main categories that essential oils fall under. Remember, since everyone interprets smells differently, this is an example and not a hard and fast rule.

- Floral (i.e. Lavender, Neroli, Jasmine)

- Woodsy (i.e. Pine, Cedar)

- Earthy (i.e. Oak moss, Vetiver, Patchouli)

- Herbaceous (i.e. Marjoram, Rosemary, Basil)

- Minty (i.e. Peppermint, Spearmint)

- Medicinal/Camphorous (i.e. Eucalyptus, Cajaput, Tea Tree)

- Spicy (i.e. Nutmeg, Clove, Cinnamon)

- Oriental (i.e. Ginger, Patchouli)

- Citrus (i.e. Orange, Lemon, Lime)

Oils that are in the same category tend to blend well together. There are also some categories that blend better together with others. Remember, the blends you like are going to be based on your personal preference, and this is just an example of some of the blends that work well together.

- Floral essential oils blend well with spicy, citrusy, and woodsy oils.

- Woodsy essential oils typically blend well with all categories.

- Spicy and oriental essential oils tend to blend well with the florals, oriental and citrus oils. However, you need to be careful that you don't overdo the blend between spicy and oriental oils, as these are stronger scents.

- Minty oils blend well with citrus, woodsy, herbaceous and earthy essential oils.

Harmonizing Your Blend

Another consideration that you must make when you are creating your blends is the depth of each essential oil and how that is going to affect your fragrance. Perhaps you have noticed before that a fragrance tends to smell differently several hours after you first apply it. This is because some essential oils evaporate more quickly than others.

Using the analogy of a musical scale, essential oils that evaporate the quickest, typically in one to two hours, are called "top notes." Essential oils that evaporate in two to four hours are considered to be "middle notes." Essential oils that take the longest to evaporate are called "base notes." Some base notes can take anywhere from four hours to a few days to evaporate.

If you go back through the descriptions of all of the oils, we covered in this book; you will see that each was labeled with a perfumery note. You can reference those notes when you are making your aromatherapy blends.

Here is a brief look at the common classification of some of the more common essential oils.

Top Notes – Essential oils that are classified as top notes normally evaporate very fast. They tend to be scents that are light, fresh and uplifting in nature. Often these essential oils are less expensive than other essential oils. Top note essential oils are volatile, fast acting and give the first impression of a blend.

Middle Notes: The majority of essential oils fall into the category of middle notes. These notes tend to be the ones that give body to the blend and have a balancing effect. The aroma of the middle notes is often not evident immediately, and it usually takes a couple of minutes to establish their scent. Middle notes are often warm and soft fragrances.

Base Notes: Essential oils that are classified as base notes are normally very heavy and have a solid fragrance. These scents are present for a long time and slow down the evaporation of the other essential oils. These fragrances are usually intense and heady. Base notes are usually rich and relaxing and nature. Essential oils that fall into the base notes category tend to be the most expensive of all essential oils.

Creating Your Blend

Step One: Think about what you want to accomplish with you blend. For many of purposes that you can achieve with essential oils, there are many oils that you can use. Consider which fragrances you enjoy the most that will perform that task.

Step Two: When you are creating your blends, start small with a total number of around twenty drops. Keep a notebook nearby to write down how many drops of what you are adding.

Step Three: Once you have created a blend of essential oils that you are happy with, you are ready to add your carrier oil. A general rule of thumb is to add one tablespoon of your carrier to every twenty drops of essential oil. You can add more if your skin is more sensitive to essential oils, although it is not recommended to add less if you are using the blend for topical applications. If you are planning on using your blend to inhale, there is no need to add a carrier.

Some Tips

-When you are blending and storing your creations, two-milliliter amber bottles are an inexpensive choice when blending in small quantities.

- Ensure that you label all of your blends clearly. If you aren't able to label the bottle, label the bottle with a number and ensure that you list exactly what is in your blend in a notebook.

- When you begin your blending, start with a ratio of thirty percent top notes, fifty percent middle notes and twenty percent base notes.

- After you create your blend, allow it to sit for a few days before you decide if you love it or hate it. The natural chemicals in the oils will interact with one another, and the aroma can change, and usually will round out a little bit over the first few days.

- Remember that there are no hard and fast rules when it comes to blending. The lack of limits and rules that are involved are what make perfumery an art form. The tips and tricks in this chapter are simply to give you a starting point and to guide you through the blending process.

Chapter 23: Frequently Asked Questions About Essential Oils

Most of your questions have probably been answered in the previous chapters. However, this chapter has been designed to be a quick point of reference for you if you forget a piece of information, or to help clarify some of the information that we covered previously. Below you are going to find some of the most commonly asked questions that people have about essential oils, as well as the answers to these questions.

Can I Consume Essential Oils?

Generally speaking, the answer is no, you cannot consume essential oils. However, like most things, there are exceptions to this. Some high-quality essential oils companies recommend using their essential oils internally. If you purchase this quality essential oils that have usage instructions that include internal use, then it has been deemed safe.

However, if you are unsure about the quality of the oils you have purchased, or if the bottle doesn't say anything about internal use, you can contact the company and ask them what they recommend. If you are purchasing essential oils because you want to consume them internally, I recommend that you contact the company beforehand to ensure that their essential oils are safe for internal consumption.

If the oils have been deemed safe for internal consumption, there are three different ways you can take them.

- **In a Capsule:** You can purchase empty capsules online, or in your local health food store. Capsules are great for taking essential oils that would normally burn your mouth if you took them undiluted or in water.

- **Under the Tongue:** Some essential oils are best taken under the tongue. This includes essential oils that are used to aid digestion. Start with one drop and wait a few minutes. You should experience relief fairly quickly after taking essential oils under the tongue, if you feel that you need another drop, you can go ahead and add one after a few minutes.

- **In Water:** Typically, if you are going to dilute essential oils in water, the dilution is one drop of the essential oil to four ounces of water. Typically, essential oils such as lemon, orange, and peppermint go the best in water.

How Often Can I Use Essential Oils?

When you are using essential oils to treat something, it is best if you use it on an as-needed basis. The danger to using essential oils when it isn't needed is that you can build up a tolerance to the essential oil and render it ineffective.

When you are using essential oils to boost your immune system or to reduce the stress, you are going to want to use it on a daily basis. To avoid becoming sensitized to essential oils, I recommend choosing a couple of essential oils that will do what you want them to and alternate between them.

Can I Use Essential Oils on Children?

There are some essential oils that are toxic to children if they are taken in large doses and there are some that are toxic to children if they are consumed internally, even in small doses. It is important to keep essential oils out of the reach of children and treat them as though they are medications. If you are going to use essential oils on children, there are a couple of tips you can follow.

Dilute: You can either dilute essential oils in a carrier oil, or you can dilute them in the bath.

Applying Topically: When you are applying essential oils to children, it is recommended to apply them to the bottom of their feet. The reason for this is that essential oils are still going to be able to enter the bloodstream quickly, but the touch skin on the bottoms of their feet are less likely to experience any irritation.

Can I Use Essential Oils on My Pet?

Animals' skin is even more sensitive than a human's skin. As such, it is important to be extremely cautious when using essential oils on animals. It is recommended that you speak to your veterinarian before using essential oils on your pet. Below are some basic guidelines on using essential oils on animals.

Dogs: Essential oils can be used in a variety of ways for a dog, from bathing to calming the nerves through diffusion. When using essential oils on your dog, you must monitor him closely for any reactions. Essential oils should be diluted at least 25% more than you would dilute it for yourself. Finally, you should always gradually introduce essential oils to ensure that there are no reactions.

Cats: Cats are especially sensitive to essential oils. As such, you should never use oils topically on a cat. If you are dispersing oils in the air, ensure that the cat has a way to get to another room for fresh air if he needs too. The same is also true for hamsters, guinea pigs, and rabbits.

Fish: Essential oils are not water-soluble. Due to this, they would end up sticking to the fish causing a host of problems. If you are diffusing the oils in the air, they should not affect fish as long as you are not diffusing right next to your fish tank.

Birds: Birds should not ever be exposed to essential oils. This includes topically and in the air, as they are extremely sensitive.

There are some essential oils that you should never use on or around your pet. These include Anise, clove, garlic, horseradish, juniper, thyme, and wintergreen and yarrow essential oils. This list is just a list of some of the more common essential oils. Always research an essential oil before using it on or around your pet. Chamomile, eucalyptus, lavender, and myrrh are all essential oils that are considered to be safe for use around pets.

Do I Need Any Special Equipment To Use Essential Oils?

While you don't necessarily need any special equipment, there are some things that will make it easier for you when you are using essential oils and will also lead to your essential oils lasting longer.

Diffuser: A diffuser is a special machine that allows you to diffuse essential oils into the air to be used for aromatherapy. While you don't need to purchase a special diffuser to enjoy aromatherapy, there are some great diffusers available that can match your décor. There are some basic diffusers that use reeds to diffuse essential oils, and there are also some on the market that you can plug in to diffuse the smell of the essential oil faster and further into the room. It is important to consider the space you are using your diffuser in when you are making your selection.

Dropper Bottles: Dropper bottles in both four and eight-ounce sizes are great when you are making your own essential oil mixes. This will allow you to experiment with different scents while being able to store them safely. Ensure that when you purchase your dropper bottles that they come with an airtight lid in addition to the dropper lid.

Carrier Oils: A good carrier oil is essential when you are diluting your essential oils. Many people like to use different carrier oils for different applications, and the carrier oil you use comes down to your personal preferences.

Spray Bottles: When you are making essential oil mixes that you want to use as an air freshener or a cleaner, a spray bottle is essential for being able to apply the mixture to where you want it without using too much.

What Kind Of Container Should I Store My Essential Oils In?

It is important that you use only glass bottles to store your pure essentials oils in. Pure essential oils are very potent, and rubber and plastic containers can be damaged and deteriorated by pure essentials oils. This also extends to the rubber dropper lid. You must ensure to remove that dropper lid from your essential oils and replace it with an airtight lid for storage. Dark amber and cobalt blue glass bottles are the best for storing pure essential oils.

You can use plastic or aluminum when you are storing your diluted essential oils. This is because the diluted essential oils aren't as potent as the pure essential oils. For example, if you add lavender essential oil to an unscented lotion, the Lavender essential oil's capacity to infuse the lotion with its aroma is not diminished, but its capacity to damage plastic and rubber is.

295

Can Essential Oils Interact With My Prescription Medications?

If you have a disease or a medical condition, or you are taking prescription medications, you need to be cautious when you begin using essential oils. It is highly recommended that you consult with a health care professional who is experienced in essential oils before you begin using them. Seek the advice of the prescribing physician as well as a pharmacist about any potential interactions between your medications and any essential oils.

Why Are Some Essential Oils More Expensive Than Others?

Essential oils are extracted from specific plant parts, and there is often only a small amount of oil in the plant part from which the oil is taken. Some plants, such as the eucalyptus, produce a high yield of oil while other plants, such as the rose, only produces a small amount of oil. In the case of the rose, it takes thirty rose heads to produce just one drop of pure rose essential oil. This is why some oils are so expensive while other oils seem more moderately priced.

What Is The Shelf Life Of Essential Oils?

Pure essential oils do not go rancid. However, over time essential oils can oxidize, deteriorate and lose their therapeutic value and aromatic qualities. The actual lifespan of essential oils can vary greatly depending on some key factors. Since many of the factors that impact the shelf life of an essential oil begin with the planting, harvesting, distillation and initial handling and storage of the essential oil it is important to shop with essential oil suppliers that you trust.

Some of the factors that can impact the shelf life of an essential oil include:

- The composition of natural chemical constituents that are present in the essential oil;

- The method of distillation that is used;

- The conditions and the care used during the distillation process;

- The quality of the botanical used;

- The care in the bottling, storage, and handling of the essential oil but your supplier and any suppliers they get essential oils from; and

- The storage conditions of the essential oil once you have received it.

As a basic rule, almost all steam distilled essential oils have a shelf life of at least two years, and even more when they are stored properly. Tea tree, pine, and fir essential oils are the exception to the above rule and typically only have a shelf life of around twelve to eighteen months due to certain components in their natural chemical composition.

Cold pressed citrus oils have the shortest shelf life of all essential oils due to the high proportion of terpenes that are more prone to oxidization. If they were fresh when you purchased them, you could expect them to last, on average, nine to twelve months.

How Can I Maximize The Shelf Life Of My Essential Oils?

To maximize the shelf life of essential oils that you have invested in, store them in dark glass bottles, keeping their caps tightly closed. Keep your essential oils in a refrigerator or a cool, dry location away from sunlight. As you use up the essential oil from a large bottle, rebottle the essential oil in a smaller bottle. This allows you to reduce the amount of headspace, or amount of oxygen, that is in contact with the essential oil.

As a final tip to knowing the shelf life of your essential oils is to ask your supplier when your oils were distilled. A reputable supplier is going to be able to tell you at least the year and the season which will give you a good idea of how long your essential oil is going to last.

How Do I Know If My Essential Oil Has Deteriorated?

The first sign you are going to have that your essential oils are deteriorated is going to be that the aroma has changed. Your nose is going to pick up on subtle smell differences before you are going to notice any visual changes. When you are able to smell that your essential oil is beginning to deteriorate, the essential oil is still safe to use, and you should try to use it up as soon as you can to prevent waste.

The next signs that your essential oils are deteriorating is that they are going to become thicker and cloudy. When you can visually see that your essential oil is thick and cloudy, it is no longer recommended for use, as they will cause skin irritation.

How Do I Dispose Of My Essential Oils

While oxidized oils are not recommended for using topically, and aren't good to be used in a diffuser, they can still be used in cleaning supplies. Be sure that you wear gloves when you are using oxidized oils in cleaning recipes. However, you might decide that this isn't an option for you. If this is the case, you need to ensure that you are disposing of your essential oils in the correct manner.

Many consumers who purchase and store essential oils forget that essential oils are highly concentrated, flammable substances that must be treated like other hazardous materials.

Essential oils should never be disposed of down the drain or through other methods that can cause the essential oil to come into contact with water supplies, vegetation, or animals. However, placing a few drops of an essential oil down your drain to freshen it is okay and is equivalent to the quantity of essential oil that would be in a bar of soap that you would use and rinse off in the shower.

When you are disposing of essential oils, it is important to look into your community's guidelines for the proper disposal of hazardous fluid ingredients. Once you are familiar with your community's guidelines, they typically aren't difficult to follow. In many places, the procedure typically involves saturating the essential oil in an inert substance like sand and then sealing the mixture in an approved container.

Conclusion

You now know about many of the different types of essential oils that are available to you, as well as some of the most commonly used carrier oils. After reading through this book, you are aware of many of the uses that essential oils have, as well as how to utilize the oils to accomplish many different health and beauty products.

You have also learned about all of the other applications essential oils can have in your life. Remember that many of the things that use essential oils only require a few drops that make it easy to replace many of the products in your home with essential oils, and save yourself a lot of time and money.

The next thing for you to do is decide which recipe you want to try first. Remember you aren't limited to the recipes that we have provided here for you. With the information you now have on carriers and essential oils, you have the information you need to make whatever you want with your essential oils!

Thank you for getting this book, I hope it provided you with all of the information you were looking for plus some information you didn't know you were looking for.

And lastly, can I ask you for a small favor? Can you please leave a review on Amazon for this book? I would highly appreciate it!

Please go to the Amazon page here

http://amzn.to/29LxJaf and write a customer review.

Thank you and Good Luck!

Made in the USA
Middletown, DE
06 November 2020

23421046R10176